Department of Health and Social Security

Priorities for Health and Personal Social Services in England

A Consultative Document

London
Her Majesty's Stationery Office

ISBN 0 11 320654 2

FOREWORD BY THE SECRETARY OF STATE
FOR SOCIAL SERVICES

This document is about the future development of our health and personal social services. In these two fields, where demand will always outstrip our capacity to meet it, it is essential at any time to work out our priorities carefully, but at this time, when the growth of public expenditure must be severely restrained, it is all the more imperative that we should choose the right priorities and plan how they can be realised. One of the important functions of this document is to provide the detailed information that will enable the right choices to be made and effective planning to be achieved.

But it does much more than that. It embodies a major new approach to planning. One of the biggest challenges to effective democratic government is how to reconcile two potentially conflicting aims: central government must be able to establish and promote certain essential national priorities, while the local agencies of government should have the maximum scope for making their own local choices in the light of their local needs. Ever since I became Secretary of State, health authorities and local authorities have been pressing for less central intervention in day to day management, and I have readily accepted that more devolution of detailed decision-making must take place. At the same time, as the Minister responsible for the National Health Service and for guiding the personal social services, I have a duty to set national policy guidelines within which local needs can be assessed. This document seeks to meet this challenge by turning planning into a co-operative enterprise: a process in which the guidelines from the centre are related to—and influenced by—the experience of those who have to apply them in local circumstances.

That is why this is a Consultative Document. The intention is that the analysis it makes of the needs we have to meet and the choices we have to make should be extensively discussed with all those involved in translating its proposals into practice: Regional Health Authorities, Area Health Authorities, local authorities, representatives of the professions and the staff, Community Health Councils, Members of Parliament, voluntary bodies and others with a close interest in these services. I shall be ready to modify these strategic plans in the light of their views, which will be reflected in the policy and planning guidelines my Department will be issuing to health and local authorities in the Spring of next year at the beginning of the next round of local planning. And within those guidelines I shall keep central intervention to the minimum.

Choice is never easy, but choose we must. We are all of us naturally concerned to protect and promote the particular aspects of the health and social problems with which we are personally involved. We are all of us likely to find that, when the allocations of resources are made, some matters will have received a lower priority than we would like. But I hope that this document will help us to see in the round the many problems and pressures we face and will thus help us all to reach the best possible planning decisions in the months ahead.

BARBARA CASTLE
Secretary of State for Social Services

CONTENTS

INTRODUCTION AND SUMMARY

1. This Consultative Document is a new departure. It is the first time an attempt has been made to establish rational and systematic priorities throughout the health and personal social services. Such an attempt is long overdue but it is given even greater urgency by the economic limitations outlined in the White Paper on Public Expenditure up to 1979/80—the period on which this document also concentrates. The level of resources which will be available over the next few years means that difficult choices will have to be made. It is essential that they should be made in full knowledge of the facts facing the services as a whole: the likely changes in demand by different client groups; the areas where past neglect has led to serious deficiencies; the ways in which the available resources can be used to get the best return; the vital importance of joint planning. It is essential, too, that central government and those who administer the services locally should work out together what the broad priorities should be.

2. This document is only the first step in what will become a continuing process. Needs, and the strategies for meeting them, necessarily change and priorities must therefore be constantly modified. The proposed consultations may also point to better ways of presenting and discussing national strategies in the future. But the need to establish a better framework for national and local planning is obvious.

3. It is intended that the strategy outlined in this document should provide health and local authorities with a basis for their own planning work and review of priorities, starting in 1976. In the same way the regional and area plans that emerge from this process will themselves contribute to the national assessment of needs and priorities. Although the Secretary of State does not have the same direct responsibility for personal social services provided by local authorities as she does for health services, there is a similar need for feedback from local planning and the Department will be discussing with the local authority associations what information local authorities should be asked to provide about their plans for their services.

4. The White Paper on Public Expenditure has shown that, despite the standstill in public expenditure as a whole from 1976/77 to 1979/80, the Government realise the need for a continuing, though reduced, growth in the health and personal social services during this period. This growth is designed to take account of demographic changes, notably the steadily rising numbers of the elderly, and the inevitably increasing sophistication and therefore cost of medical treatment. The White Paper makes clear that there will be no further cuts in the expenditure planned for 1976/77, which will enable current expenditure on personal social services to rise by 4 per cent and on the National Health Service by 2·6 per cent. In the subsequent years the average annual rates of growth will be 2 per cent and 1·8 per cent respectively. Within the National Health Service the family practitioner services will grow at an average of 3·7 per cent a year from 1975/76 to 1979/80.

5. These figures face those responsible for these services with two challenges: first, the figures are much lower than in recent years and so former plans will have to be re-assessed but, secondly, the figures still contain an element of growth which allows a margin for manoeuvre and for the development of new

iatives. This has made it possible for the Secretary of State to implement important aspects of her policies in the health services: the redistribution of resources in favour of the deprived regions and areas; and the encouragement of joint planning between health authorities and local authorities through the provision of special finance. One of the lessons to emerge from the analysis in this document is the crucial importance of joint planning by health and local authorities of their provision for those groups, like the mentally handicapped, where their responsibilities so clearly overlap. In order to encourage the establishment of joint care planning teams their work is now backed by the provision of resources specially allotted for this purpose. The Department is discussing with local authorities and health authorities the detailed arrangements for this joint financing for which sums rising to £27m by 1979/80 are proposed in the document.

6. When resources are limited it is clear that growth in any particular service can only be afforded if counterbalancing economies are made elsewhere. The document reviews each service in detail, and suggests that authorities, in the planning decisions they have to make in the next few months, should be guided by the following order of priorities.

7. The first essential is to maintain the standard of services: to put people before buildings. Within the overall increase in the programmes, capital expenditure will be cut back in order to allow current expenditure to rise from 1976/77 by 1·8 per cent a year for the National Health Service and 2 per cent a year for the personal social services. Though rationalisation may mean changes in the patterns of provision and some concentration of facilities in the interests of greater efficiency, the standard of service should in general be maintained. The capital programme for health services, which for England will level out at about £250m a year (including by 1979/80 £15m allotted for joint financing) will still allow a modest number of major hospital schemes of high priority to proceed, in addition to improvements in existing buildings. But the document emphasises the importance of concentrating on low cost projects wherever possible and on innovations, such as the nucleus hospital.

8. Personal social services capital expenditure is projected to level out at £44m which will be supplemented by joint finance capital. This should enable some development of services for the elderly and the younger physically handicapped, children, and the mentally ill and handicapped.

9. The document restates the role of primary care in helping to relieve pressure on hospital and residential services by caring for more people in the community. The family practitioner services will continue to expand, at an average of 3·7 per cent a year; the health centre programme will be maintained and it is proposed that the growth of vital supporting services such as health visitors and home nursing should be given high priority. An expansion of 6 per cent a year in both these services is visualised.

10. It is also important to avoid false economies. There should be increasing emphasis on preventive services. It is proposed that the health education programme should be preserved, and that expenditure on family planning should increase. A key element in the proposed strategy is to maintain and where necessary increase the level of training and to improve the ways in which skilled manpower is used. For example, the expansion of vocational training for family

doctors will be pressed ahead, and allowance is made for the first phase of implementing recommendations in the report—which is shortly to be published —of the Working Party on Manpower and Training for the Social Services. The Government intend to introduce legislation for the implementation of two major reports on the training of health professions—the Briggs report on nurse training, and the Merrison report on the regulation of the medical profession.

11. The document also highlights two problems: the extent of unsatisfied need in the provision for the mentally ill and the mentally handicapped and the pressure on services due to the rising numbers of elderly and of children, or families with children, needing help. It therefore suggests that unless the targets for meeting these needs are to be abandoned, there must be a deliberate decision to give them priority over the development of the general and acute hospital services; and that there should be some reduction in expenditure on maternity services, where in recent years costs have risen in spite of a falling birthrate. Within the overall growth rate of just over 2 per cent for current expenditure over the years 1975/76-1979/80, the following average rates of increase for major service groupings would be necessary to fulfil the priorities set out in the document.

> Services used mainly by the *elderly* (and in some instances by younger physically handicapped people)—including hospital geriatric provision, home nursing, residential homes, day care, home helps and meals— 3·2 per cent a year.
>
> Services for the *mentally ill* (hospital provision, local authority residential and day care provision) 1·8 per cent a year.
>
> Services for the *mentally handicapped* (hospital provision, local authority residential and day care provision) 2·8 per cent a year.
>
> Services mainly for children and families with children: 2·2 per cent a year.
>
> Acute and general hospital services: 1·2 per cent a year.
>
> Expenditure on the hospital maternity services would fall by 1·8 per cent a year.

12. Such a pattern of distribution would broadly maintain the rate of progress towards the targets set out in the White Paper of 1971 on the Mentally Handicapped and the recent White Paper on Mental Illness. The elderly would benefit from the emphasis on community services and the aim of releasing acute hospital facilities for geriatric use. The phasing out of pay-beds from NHS hospitals will increase the number of acute beds available to NHS patients, and the scope for using acute beds for the elderly will be increased. The level of growth proposed for the acute services would pose serious problems that can only be overcome through the rationalisation of the services: by, for example, the development of day-surgery units and five-day wards, and by reducing the length of in-patient stay in areas where it is markedly higher than elsewhere. The potential savings here are estimated at between £20m and £40m.

13. If this pattern is followed the shares of total expenditure (capital as well as current) that would result for each programme are as shown at Figure 1. On this basis the shares for mental handicap, mental illness, the elderly and primary care will all rise. The share for children's services would be about the same and

3

the shares for general and acute hospital services and the maternity services would fall. The shares of current expenditure alone are shown at Figure 2.

14. If the strategy suggested is to succeed, all parts of the services must make their contribution to economies. Members of the medical profession, while preserving their clinical freedom, must be ready to seek more economical methods of providing health services which will enable the available resources to be used more efficiently and in some cases freed for other purposes. The drug bill of the NHS has been growing at 5 per cent a year and is expected to continue growing at this rate. It is essential that unnecessarily lavish prescribing should be avoided. It is also important to develop procurement policies for medical equipment and other supplies for the NHS that will give better guidance on purchases and strengthen the production base of the medical equipment industry. Proposals to this end are being discussed with the professions and the health authorities. With clinical and field services under such severe restraint it is obvious that there must be a searching review of administrative overheads, which has already been set in hand.

Form of document

15. Section I describes recent trends in the development of the services as a whole, deals with future resources in more detail than this introduction and highlights the main theatres in the suggested campaign for a more economical approach. Section II deals briefly with the general implications for staff of the suggested strategy. Sections III-X describe in detail the recent development and the suggested priorities for each main group of services; and the staffing implications will no doubt be an important element in the national and local consultations. Each of these sections begins with a short summary of its contents. The concluding Section XI deals briefly with the development of the services after 1980.

Summary of method

16. The detailed proposals in Sections III-X would give effect to the general priorities we have outlined. In each section, the future priority suggested for each service is illustrated by annual growth rates in current expenditure between 1975/76 and 1979/80. The different growth rates suggested for each service are summarised in Tables 1 and 2 of Annex 2 (pages 82 and 83). All expenditure figures are at 1975 public expenditure survey prices (the price base for which is November 1974) and therefore reflect past and suggested changes in the volume of real resources. They are based on a "programme budget" developed in the Department for costing policies. Apart from the general and acute hospital services, and the primary care services (including the family practitioner services) which, generally speaking, may be used by the whole community, services are considered from the standpoint of the various client groups by which they are mainly used. For example, hospital geriatric provision, local authority residential homes and day centres used mainly by old people, the home nursing service, the chiropody service, home helps and the local authority meals service, are brought together as "Services used mainly by the elderly". Broad groupings have been chosen to facilitate links with field planning (which will be mainly in service terms), but at the same time to enable the various services to be viewed as they affect the main client groups who use them. Details of the method are given in Annex 2.

17. The figures are approximate and relate to the services viewed nationally. The purposes of giving the suggested growth rates up to 1979/80 are to illustrate the different degrees of priority which are suggested for each service and to show how these relative priorities might be implemented within the total resources available. The Department has in the past been criticised for advocating priorities without proper regard to their expenditure implications and without showing which services should be held back to accommodate them. The consultative document is in part designed as a response to this criticism. Local priorities will naturally be affected by a range of factors—demographic, social and practical—peculiar to individual areas; and it is accepted that local plans will often not correspond to the order of national priorities proposed here.

18. There are also some general points to be made. The first is that many of the policies set out in detail in the sections dealing with particular services are already generally established and accepted. For mental illness and mental handicap, for example, the direction of advance has been mapped out in White Papers. It is on the balance of priority between these policies, rather than on the policies themselves, that we are primarily inviting views.

19. In projecting forward the effect of continuing these policies we do not intend to stifle worthwhile innovations. The impetus for development of policies has in the past come from the conception and testing out by individuals of new methods of treatment and patterns of care, which, when they have proved themselves, the Department has helped to promote. Our aim will be to allow maximum scope for local innovation and individual initiatives which can improve services within the resources available.

20. A review of priorities across the health and personal social services has to be comprehensive, but as brief as possible. The selection of points to be mentioned has been a difficult compromise between these aims. In subsequent documents giving guidelines on national priorities, it should be possible for the Department to deal with the issues more briefly by reference back to this document. Suggestions for dealing with particular issues in greater detail will be discussed during the consultation period.

Expenditure by programme as a percentage of Total Expenditure
Current & Capital Expenditure (£m November 1974 prices)

Figure 1

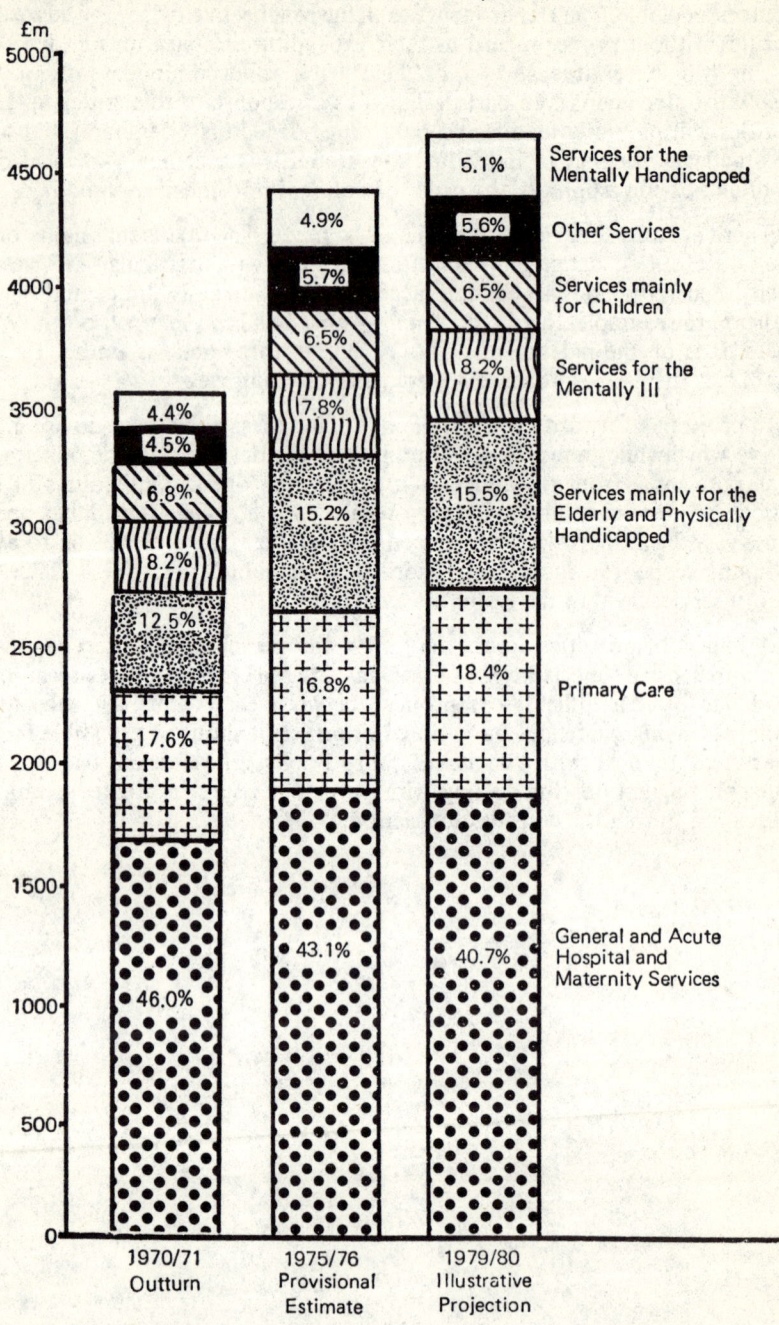

£m

Expenditure by programme as a percentage of Total Expenditure   Figure 2
Current Expenditure (£m November 1974 prices)

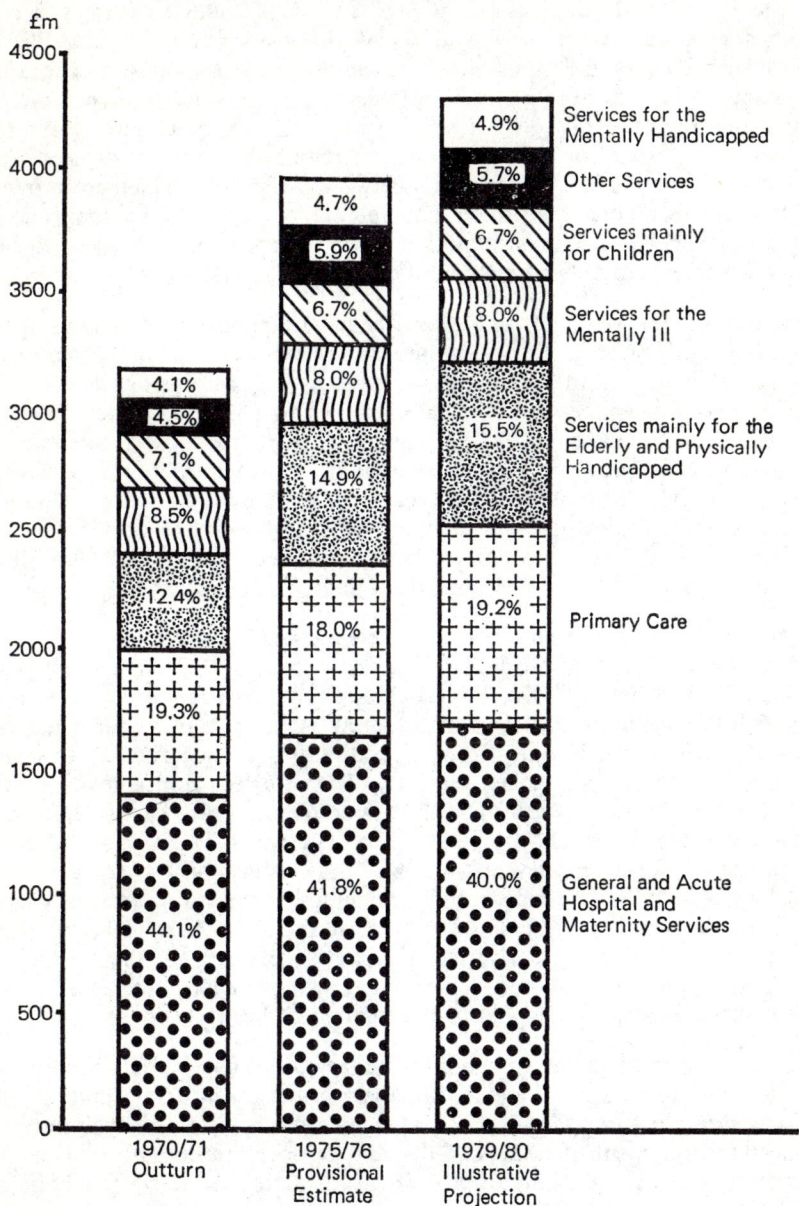

I

THE SERVICES AS A WHOLE: RECENT DEVELOPMENTS, PRESENT PRESSURES, AND FUTURE RESOURCES

1.1 The health and personal social services (HPSS) aim to meet the community's need for health care and social support as fully as possible. As knowledge advances and skills improve, the services are able to do more and the public expects more to be done. Standards of need tend to be relative and what is reasonable at any given time depends on what the country can afford and is willing to pay for as well as on professional assessments of need. As a result there is always likely to be a gap between the services which are provided and the demands made upon them. Difficult choices have to be made to decide how far particular demands should be met. These choices are particularly hard when there can only be a slow rate of growth in resources.

1.2 In the last few years nearly all services have expanded. The expansion has been particularly large in the community care services which aim to help people to live an independent life in their own homes as long as possible. The aim has been to enable hospitals and residential homes to admit only those who are temporarily or permanently unable to manage at home or who need services which cannot be properly provided or which it would be too expensive to provide at home. This trend towards care in the community has been encouraged by recent legislation which has required local authorities to provide services to certain groups (the Local Authority Social Services Act, the Chronically Sick and Disabled Persons Act, and the Children and Young Persons Act).

1.3 The expansion has been made possible by a steady growth in the resources used by the services over the last twelve and particularly the last seven years. Between 1968/69 and 1974/75 the population grew by 0·2 per cent a year on average but expenditure on the services grew at the rate of about 4 per cent a year in real terms. For health services the growth rate was 3 per cent a year but for the personal social services, which started from a relatively low base, it was 10 per cent a year. The shift to community care has brought rapid expansion of the local authority personal social services. The biggest increase—an average of 14 per cent a year—followed the establishment of social services departments in 1971. The most rapidly expanding services (in terms of current expenditure) have been residential, day care and domiciliary services which are used mainly by the elderly, the physically handicapped, the mentally ill and handicapped and children. There have also been large increases in day patient facilities at hospitals and in the number of health centres.

1.4 The expansion and development of the services in recent years has enabled considerable progress to be made, but the services taken as a whole are still under severe pressure. This is illustrated by waiting lists and waiting times for hospital treatment, pressures of demand on local authority social services departments, and the difficulty of providing satisfactory services where buildings are obsolete.

1.5 There is also a need progressively to remedy the large variations in standards between different regions, areas, and districts. For example, by the crude measure of expenditure per head of population, regional variations ranged as follows in 1972:—

	Highest Region	*Lowest Region*
Hospital services	£37·19	£21·09
Family Practitioner Services	£11·45	£9·20
Personal Social Services	£8·78	£5·12

How far these variations reflect differences in need is not known for certain; but there are clearly major inequities in the distribution of services which must be corrected.

Future increases in demand

Population projections

1.6 The projections made by the Office of Population Censuses and Surveys based on the estimated mid-1974 population are as follows:—

HOME POPULATION IN ENGLAND—MILLIONS

	1973	1979	1985	% change 1971–1973	% change 1973–1979	% change 1973–1985
Children under 5	3·5	2·8	3·5	− 4	−19	0
Children 5–15	8·1	7·9	6·8	+ 3	− 3	−17
Adults 16–64	28·4	28·8	29·8	0	+ 1	+ 5
Elderly 65–74	4·1	4·3	4·1	+ 4	+ 5	− 1
Elderly 75+	2·3	2·5	2·8	+ 3	+13	+25
Total	46·4	46·4	47·0	+ 1	0	+ 1
All Births	0·6	0·6	0·8	−14	− 1	+20

(Note: Discrepancies are due to rounding.)

These trends are illustrated in the chart at Annex 1. They show little change in the total population but considerable changes in the numbers in different age groups. The birth rate, which has been falling over the last few years, is projected to rise as women born between the mid-1950s and mid-1960s start to have their children. By 1985 it is expected that:—

– the number of births will be back at about the 1969 level
– the number of children under five will be back at the 1973 level
– there will be over a million less children under 16 than in 1973
– there will be half a million more elderly people over 75 than in 1973.

1.7 While the projections of the numbers of births and of young children are necessarily uncertain, those of the number of elderly people are relatively reliable. The expected increase in the elderly is particularly important as they make heavy demands on hospitals and residential homes and on most social work, primary health, and community care services.

1.8 Movements of population between regions are expected to continue. There has been a particularly high rate of migration of people of working age to the East Midlands and East Anglia, and of retired people to East Anglia and the South West.

Rising standards of care and treatment

1.9 Developments in medical science, innovations in methods of treatment, and the development of new patterns of community care are all major influences on demand for resources. Pressures for improvements and expansion come from staff, professional bodies, the public and the Department itself. In the last few years, there has been particular concern about standards of care for the elderly, the physically handicapped, the mentally ill and handicapped, and children whose families cannot provide a satisfactory environment for them. These pressures are likely to increase the demands made on the services.

Future resources—The general economic background

1.10 The Government have made clear that for some years at any rate public expenditure will need to be constrained in the national economic interest. In the annual White Paper on Public Expenditure published in February (Cmnd 6393), the Government explain their strategy for public expenditure in the years up to and including 1979/80 (the period covered most fully in this document).

1.11 The White Paper begins by explaining that two problems stand out in the management of total public spending:—

"The first has been with us for many years. Popular expectations for improved public services and welfare programmes have not been matched by the growth in output—or by willingness to forego improvements in private living standards in favour of those programmes. The oil crisis intensified this gap between expectations and available resources. The second problem is that of cost inflation, which has become acute in the last few years, and has added an extra dimension of difficulty".

1.12 At a time of world recession public expenditure can help us to sustain employment, with a consequent high public sector deficit; but as demand picks up resources must be freed for exports and investment. The Government's plans therefore include no further cuts in public expenditure in 1976/77: indeed some additional provision is being made to help deal with unemployment in the short term. But the programmes for 1977/78 onwards shown in the previous White Paper (Cmnd 5879, published in January 1975) have been substantially revised in order:—

"– first, to stabilise the total level of spending on the expenditure programmes for the time being, so that enough resources are available for increased exports and investment;
– second, to give priority to expenditure for improving industrial productivity and efficiency, and hence to increase the rate of growth of resources."

1.13 This strategy is explained in the White Paper as follows:
"The programmes in Cmnd 5879 provided for some continuing growth of expenditure during this period. In order to stabilise the level of spending, the total size of those programmes in that White Paper has been scaled down. . . . As soon as a sound economic base can be achieved, some growth in spending should again be possible. But at least during the next three years or so, no overall growth in public expenditure (excluding debt interest) is planned beyond the level now envisaged for 1976/77. This means that in all programmes, including the social programmes, very strict tests of priority have had to be applied. The Government's purpose in making these hard decisions was to ensure that the increase in national

output in the next three or four years is not appropriated for use in the public sector, but instead is available to put the balance of payments right, to provide increased productive investment, and to allow a modest rate of increase in private consumption. Holding public expenditure and public service manpower broadly steady while output increases will permit that shift of resources which it is their strategic aim to bring about."

HPSS resources to 1979/80

1.14 As explained in the Introduction, the effect of the White Paper allocations is that between 1976/77 and 1979/80, personal social services' *current* expenditure will rise by 2 per cent a year and National Health Service current expenditure by 1·8 per cent a year. Between 1975/76 and 1976/77, the rates of increase are higher—4 per cent and 2·6 per cent respectively.

1.15 If health and local authorities jointly agree to use the sums proposed for joint financing over the period (£12m current expenditure and £15m capital expenditure in 1979/80), the scope for additional expenditure on community services for the elderly, the physically handicapped, the mentally ill and the mentally handicapped will be increased. The growth of personal social services' current expenditure between 1976/77 and 1979/80 will be 2 per cent a year, but there will be a potential additional growth of ½ per cent a year for jointly financed community social services. Without this additional growth, the highly desirable switch from hospital services to community care throughout this period will be greatly reduced, and it would be impossible to envisage keeping to the long-term strategies set out in the White Papers *Better Services for the Mentally Ill* and *Better Services for the Mentally Handicapped*.

1.16 A reduction in *capital* expenditure will be necessary both to ensure that adequate provision is made for current expenditure and to relate the size of capital investment to the ability to meet the additional current costs to which it gives rise. If health and local authorities jointly agree to use for community social services the allocation of joint finance capital (rising to £15m in 1979/80), hospital and community health capital expenditure in 1979/80 will be about £235m, and personal social services' capital about £59m.

1.17 It is recognised that many much needed new hospitals and other developments will not be able to proceed within these totals, and the size of other projects will have to be reduced and their timetables extended. However, there should be scope for the completion of schemes under construction, and a modest programme of new developments of high priority, together with schemes needed to maintain existing services—for example the replacement of medical equipment, ambulances and engineering plant.

General priorities, and the need for economy

1.18 The projected levels of capital expenditure and the rate of growth of current expenditure are considerably lower than in recent years. This has been made necessary by the economic outlook, but the Government have given the HPSS a considerable priority by allocating some resources for growth within their overall strategy of stabilising the level of public expenditure after 1976/77.

1.19 The challenge to those who plan, manage, and work in the services is to find ways of developing them over the next few years so that the most urgent needs are met, whether they arise from the increasing number of elderly people, or from the need to overcome past neglect by implementing new policies (for example mental illness, mental handicap and services for children), or from pressures for the introduction of improved techniques and patterns of providing care.

1.20 The suggested priorities for developing particular services are summarised in the Introduction. The proposals would enable some limited progress to be made towards developing the services concerned, by using the "growth money" as far as possible on services of first priority—notably those for the elderly and physically handicapped, the mentally ill and handicapped, and children. We suggest that they should be regarded as a minimum, and that every effort should be made to achieve further improvements in these and other services by exploiting fully such scope as there may be for economies and rationalisation. In particular all concerned should:—

- use *low cost solutions* wherever this can be done without damage to standards of care, whether in new developments or by substitution in existing services;
- review the *level of provision* in all services, with a view to finding particular elements which can be reduced in current circumstances. Some services may have been justified when they were first established, but changes in the patterns of need and provision may mean that the resources could be used more efficiently elsewhere.

1.21 No service should be exempt from this review, but two areas are of particular importance—general administration costs, and the general and acute hospital services. The identifiable costs of administration account for a relatively small proportion of HPSS expenditure, and good administrative and supporting services make a major contribution to the standard and cost-effectiveness of care and treatment given directly to the community. Good management can save money, and the demands on it are greater in a period of financial constraint. There is however a particular responsibility on management in all parts of the services, and in the Department, to ensure that it carries out its own activities efficiently and economically. The Secretary of State has already advised health authorities that the creation and filling of any additional administrative posts and the filling of vacancies should not take place until both the need for a post relative to the specific job of work and the real priority of the work have been fully considered. She is also discussing with health authorities and staff representatives the guidelines for a review of the scope for economies in administration.

1.22 Of particular importance is a review of general and acute hospital and maternity services because this is the largest block of expenditure (some 40 per cent of the total) and because these services probably offer the greatest scope for redeployment of resources. There has already been a good deal of redeployment of resources in these fields largely due to scrutiny, by the medical profession in particular, of clinical priorities and methods. There is no question of interfering in clinical decisions but a realistic review of service priorities must involve discussion with the professions of the extent to which resources can be released by further developments of this kind. We review the scope for this in Section IV. We recognise that the acute hospital services themselves face

12

serious problems—for example waiting lists and waiting times, the growing number of elderly patients and the need to introduce new methods of treatment. The challenge here will be to make the patterns of existing provision more efficient in resource terms, so that the improvements can be funded from internal savings, and, in some localities at least, some resources can be transferred to other local programmes and services.

Voluntary organisations

1.23 In the coming years, the contributions—of time, ideas, and money—that people in the community voluntarily make to the running of the services will be more than ever important. Health and local authorities should give every support to voluntary bodies in their work of harnessing community effort. The Department will be maintaining its support for national voluntary bodies.

Geographical reallocation of resources

1.24 The changes in resource deployment implied in these strategies are fairly marginal, though their achievement will require consistent efforts by all concerned. Following the work of the Resource Allocation Working Party, in which Departmental and health authority officials considered means of distributing NHS funds more equitably between regions, there is also to be a shift of resources towards those regions and localities which, historically, have received less funds per head of population than others, and where standards of service have suffered accordingly. Regions and localities which receive restricted allocations on this account will need to conduct a particularly searching review of their services, so that those services which are relatively well provided with facilities and staff can yield resources to those which are underdeveloped.

IMPLICATIONS FOR STAFF

2.1 There will need to be careful consultation—both locally and nationally—on the implications of the proposed priorities for staff, but it is not expected that there will be any general problems of manpower shortage or redundancy. However, since over 70 per cent of HPSS current expenditure is on staff, the recent rapid growth in overall staff numbers cannot continue. It will also be necessary for some staff to be redeployed, with their agreement, so that the new priorities can be achieved.

2.2 By encouraging a more participative style of management and more effective mechanisms for consultation at local and national levels, industrial relations can be improved, within existing resources, so as to help in carrying out these tasks. A number of initiatives on these lines are already in train. Staff at all levels can make a major contribution to improving the running of the services. Moreover staff should be involved at all levels in the search for economies and for better ways of using resources, so that the maximum possible improvements can be made in services to patients within the limited growth that is available.

2.3 There are two other matters of long-term importance to NHS staff—their role in the direct management of authorities, and the Whitley Council system. As the Secretary of State announced on 11 July 1975 the membership of each Regional and Area Health Authority is to be extended to include, in addition to the two doctors and one nurse or midwife already serving, two other members drawn from those serving in the NHS. Consultations are currently taking place about how these new members should be elected. And in April 1975 the Secretary of State appointed Dr McCarthy (now Lord McCarthy of Headington) as a part-time adviser in industrial relations with the specific task of reviewing the working of the NHS Whitley machinery. He is expected to report in the summer.

Training and facilities for staff

2.4 The skills and commitment of staff are the services' most important asset. Standards of treatment and care are largely set by the caring professions themselves, but they need to be supported by training and good staff management.

2.5 It is more than ever important that training should be rigorously examined for its continued relevance and effectiveness, but it would be a false economy to make any general cutback in training programmes. Well-designed training programmes can make a very significant contribution to enhanced efficiency and flexibility in the use of resources and deployment of staff without which the strategies we suggest for the services will be unattainable. It will be important within the limited resources available to make room for training of this kind.

2.6 As regards particular training programmes, it is intended that the momentum behind existing arrangements for the vocational training of general medical practitioners, and for the in-service training of other skilled groups such as nurses, should be maintained. In addition training opportunities for developing new types of skill (such as the specialty of community medicine) should be maintained and developed.

2.7 Certain groups, however, have particularly urgent training needs. For social workers and other social services personnel an expansion of training is a particularly important priority, as is recognised in the report of the Working Party on Manpower and Training for the Social Services which is shortly to be published.

2.8 For nurses, it is important to retain over the country as a whole at least the existing level of resources devoted to training, and in due course there will need to be a substantial increase in order to implement the recommendations of the Briggs Report on nurse training. The need for legislation (preparation of which is continuing) means that in any event implementation could probably not begin in earnest much before 1979 or 1980. However, the annual cost once the new style of training has been fully introduced is estimated to be £27m. It would be very difficult to accommodate this within the growth available to the HPSS up to 1979/80. The timing of full implementation will need to be discussed against other priorities, and the consultative proposal is that it should be one of the first priorities if there is a higher growth rate after 1979/80.

2.9 The Government place a very high priority on the achievement of a medical school student intake of some 4,000 a year by 1980, which will enable a higher proportion of posts in hospitals and general practice to be filled by British graduates. It is important that sufficient pre-registration posts should be available for this increased output. The NHS must aim to make the best use of these young doctors, and give them full opportunity for adequate post-graduate training. This need not add much to total costs, but will require some reorganisation of posts, especially to provide suitable training for women graduates with domestic commitments.

2.10 The requirements of the Health and Safety at Work Act and other employment legislation will need to be met. Other developments which of themselves would be desirable will, however, have to be deferred. It is, for example, unlikely that significant expansion in occupational health services will be possible for the time being. Here as in similar fields the aim must be to ensure that money already being spent is well spent.

PRIMARY CARE, COMMUNITY HEALTH AND PREVENTION

The primary care services are largely conditioned by the type and level of patient demand on the family practitioner services. To meet the estimated increase in demand for these services, particularly the extension of family planning and primary care for the elderly, and to cover the rising cost of the pharmaceutical bill, provision has been made for expenditure on the primary care services as a whole to rise by about 3·8 per cent a year.

Emphasis should be given to:—

- encouraging the development of primary health care teams, and where necessary, to encouraging a better distribution of manpower. The proposal to maintain a relatively large health centre capital programme should assist in this;

- giving priority to preventive activities and family planning services;

- preventing pharmaceutical costs from rising unduly, and securing better value for expenditure on drugs.

3.1 These services include the general medical, dental, ophthalmic, and pharmaceutical services, health centres and clinics, family planning outside the hospital service, and preventive activities in the community including vaccination, immunisation and fluoridation. Their current cost is about £720m of which about £310m is spent on the pharmaceutical services, and £370m on other family practitioner services. They are to a large extent provided by independent contractors from their own premises and do not involve much NHS capital expenditure. Capital expenditure by NHS authorities in 1975/76 was about £24m, nearly all spent on health centres.

3.2 Home nursing, health visiting, much ante- and post-natal care, and chiropody are an integral part of the primary care services. All have an important role in preventive measures designed to maintain health and keep people out of hospitals. They are used mainly by particular groups of patients (for example the elderly and the physically handicapped and children), and are discussed further in Sections V and IX (where it is suggested, for example, that health visiting and home nursing services should both be expanded by 6 per cent a year).

3.3 Family practitioners are normally the patient's first point of contact with the NHS. They give all the care needed in the great majority of illnesses. Their main objectives, with the support of other members of the primary health care team—particularly health visitors and home nurses—are to promote health and prevent disease and disability, and to provide care for patients who do not require the often expensive facilities and specialist services of hospitals. The preventive role of the primary care team is fulfilled generally through advice to patients as well as specifically through, for example, immunisation and vaccination.

3.4 The primary care services are provided in two ways—by practitioners who enter into contracts for services with Family Practitioner Committees, and by other professional staff employed by Area Health Authorities. For the most part the primary care services are conditioned by the level and type of patient demand, and by the individual professional decisions of the independent contractors who provide them. Though future expenditure on them can be broadly forecast, it is not susceptible to the same degree of budgetary control as expenditure on services directly provided by the statutory field authorities. The practitioner services are directly financed by the Department through the Family Practitioner Committees, and (except for AHA-employed nurses and health visitors who work with family doctors) their costs are not a charge on health authority budgets.

3.5 It would be difficult to extend close budgetary control to expenditure on the practitioner services and undesirable at a time when changes in the pattern of hospital provision (for example, earlier patient discharge) may have implications for the role of primary care. In general it is not proposed to intervene in the natural development of the primary care services, as determined by demand and professional response to it. On this basis it is forecast that expenditure on the family practitioner services (including pharmaceutical costs) will increase by about 3·7 per cent a year between 1975/76 and 1979/80. This increase should make possible some reduction in referral to the hospital services where this can be achieved without detriment to patient care. On the community side, where services are provided directly by AHAs, a broadly comparable increase is assumed, largely attributable to the development of family planning services.

3.6 The main objectives suggested for the next few years are :—

   – to encourage the development of primary health care teams in order to:

      (a) improve the preventive and curative services in the community;

      (b) allow for the increased workload which will result from the greater number of old people;

      (c) reduce demands on the acute hospital services.

   – to remedy persistent shortages of personnel in localities where they occur, by encouraging a better distribution of manpower;

   – to prevent pharmaceutical costs from rising unduly and secure better value from expenditure on drugs;

   – to give priority to preventive measures and family planning services.

General medical practice and associated primary health care teams

3.7 Recent developments have included:—

   – an average increase in the number of doctors providing the full range of medical services of about 300 (1½ per cent) a year between 1970 and 1974;

   – a substantial increase over the same period in the numbers of health visitors—an average of 340 (over 4 per cent) a year—and of home nurses— an average of 550 (nearly 6 per cent) a year;

   – a considerable increase in the last five years in the number of health centres: only 124 were opened between 1948 and 1969, but since then there have been a further 453, and about 15 per cent of general practitioners now practise from them;

- an increasing tendency for family doctors to work in groups (about 60 per cent of them now belong to practices with three or more doctors) and in conjunction with other health professions (some 80 per cent of home nurses and health visitors are now attached to general medical practices). In some areas, social workers employed by local authorities are also attached to primary health care teams.

- the expansion of voluntary post-registration vocational training for entrants to general practice.

- agreement (as from July 1975) of the terms of service under which family doctors may provide family planning services to women patients;

- continued concentration on health education and preventive health in the training of health visitors and increasing emphasis on these aspects in the training arrangements for home nurses.

3.8 The family doctor services and primary health care teams will be affected, as will all other services, by the need for economies. Some desirable developments will have to be foregone—for example a new and significantly improved system of medical records has had to be deferred. However, the continued expansion and improvement of these services should be a high priority.

3.9 The growth of 6 per cent a year for home nurses and health visitors employed by health authorities but working in collaboration with family doctors should lead to a considerable development of primary health care teams. We estimate that the number of family doctors will continue to rise broadly in accordance with recent trends. The vocational training of entrants to general practice is one of the best ways of improving the quality of the primary medical services. The cost is relatively small, and the training programme already well established. It is intended to keep up the momentum of the programme.

3.10 Health centres make an important contribution to the development of primary care teamwork. In spite of the general need to reduce capital expenditure, we propose that a substantial programme (£17m in 1979/80) should be maintained. This is somewhat lower than the expenditure of £23m estimated for 1975/76, but the programme in 1975/76 has been larger than in recent years. Priority should be given to establishing health centres in areas where inadequate accommodation is hampering the development of primary care teams.

3.11 Taking account of the estimated increase in the number of family doctors, the increase in the elderly population (the capitation fee for elderly patients is higher than for others) and the rising cost of family planning services, it is forecast that the cost of general medical practice will rise by about 3 per cent a year. The cost of prescriptions by family doctors is forecast to rise at a higher rate, and the annual increase suggested for the home nursing and health visiting services is higher still (6 per cent a year).

3.12 The degree of priority given to primary medical care and its associated expenditure is thus higher than for any other group of services of comparable size, and it can be achieved only by restraining growth in other services. It is therefore of great importance that expenditure on primary medical care should be fully cost effective, so that it yields the largest possible benefits to the community, and enables the burdens on other services (where growth is more limited) to be lightened to the extent that this is feasible.

3.13 The fullest co-operation of individual family doctors holds the key to achieving value for money, and discussions will take place with their representatives, and with other bodies concerned, on five main issues:—

- the recruitment and distribution of family doctors;

- training requirements in the light of the Government's commitment to vocational training;

- the need to improve the flow of pharmaceutical information to doctors, and for more effective prescription monitoring (see paragraph 3.18 below);

- the need to maintain the impetus towards health care teams, particularly in deprived areas, in the light of the high priority given within the capital programme to health centre building;

- the need to exercise a better control of deputising services in the interests of patient care.

General dental and ophthalmic services

3.14 In these services both the overall net cost and the level of demand are affected by the charges payable by patients, as well as by the number and distribution of practitioners and the range of NHS services which they are willing to provide. In the *general dental services* there has been a growth in the number of practitioners of about $1-1\frac{1}{2}$ per cent a year over the past five years. This is expected to continue. The number of courses of dental treatment continues also to rise. Maldistribution of general dental services remains a cause of concern. After full discussion an experimental new scheme will be introduced on a small scale initially. This will involve remunerating dentists by salary plus incentive bonuses and the provision of premises and equipment by Area Health Authorities. The scheme will be offered in localities where it is difficult to obtain NHS dental treatment.

3.15 On the hypothesis that the overall yield of charges to patients for dental treatment will remain at a constant proportion of the total costs of the treatment given, the net cost of the general dental service is estimated to rise by about 2 per cent a year to 1979/80.

3.16 On the same hypothesis about charges, the net costs of the *general ophthalmic services* will rise by about 3 per cent a year to 1979/80. Growth of this order would broadly reflect the trend in recent years for the number of sight tests and spectacles supplied to increase, partly as a result of the growth in the elderly population.

Pharmaceutical services

3.17 These services account for the largest block of primary care expenditure, and their cost has been growing at about 5 per cent a year. It is forecast that up to 1979/80 growth of about this order will continue. This forecast assumes that prescription charges will remain at the same cash level as they are now so that in real terms their value will progressively reduce. It also assumes that the number of prescriptions will continue to rise; that their average cost will increase as a result of the introduction of more advanced preparations; and that there will be an increase in the number of family planning prescriptions.

However, it is not envisaged that in a period of severe restraint on HPSS resources any significant additional expenditure would be incurred as a result of deliberate extensions of the pharmaceutical services.

3.18 In an attempt to secure good value for money on pharmaceutical expenditure proposals have been put to the industry and the professions about costs and methods of promotion, and means of improving educational information given to prescribers. The aim is to reduce the emphasis on promotion (for most of which the NHS ultimately pays) and to put greater stress on good quality information for prescribers because their individual decisions influence the cost and determine the efficiency of drug use.

Community health, the preventive services, and the promotion of health

3.19 The financial projections include expenditure for certain specific community health and preventive services. These items are:—

family planning (ie in clinics inherited from local authorities in 1974) at an estimated total cost in 1975/76 of £12m. An additional £3m has been allocated for 1975/76 for sterilisation in hospital; this is included in the general and acute hospital programme;

health education, vaccination, immunisation, fluoridation and other specific preventive activities; in 1975/76 expenditure on this block of activities was estimated at about £15m.

Family planning

3.20 Family planning will continue to develop and a further increase of about £2m is projected by 1979/80 after which it is assumed that the expenditure will remain stable. The rates of growth of the family planning clinic services and the general practitioner family planning services are interdependent. The working groups established within each health district in accordance with paragraph 7 of the Department's circular HSC(IS)32 can assist in the preparation of integrated plans for developing family planning in each locality.

Vaccination and immunisation

3.21 It is also important that the vaccination and immunisation programmes should be maintained and where possible strengthened. There is a risk that the success of the programmes in combating many of the main infectious diseases, especially those of childhood, may lead to a false sense of security. Care should be taken not to lose ground that has been hard won over many years.

Fluoridation

3.22 A recent report of the Royal College of Physicians has further confirmed the benefits to dental health of fluoridated water supply and has shown that there are no health risks associated with it. The Government have consequently renewed their recommendation to health authorities. To encourage authorities to spend the relatively small amount of capital required, £0·5m a year is to be earmarked for authorities wishing to proceed with fluoridation schemes.

Other preventive measures

3.23 But the specific preventive measures covered as separate items in the financial projections are only a small part of preventive effort as a whole.

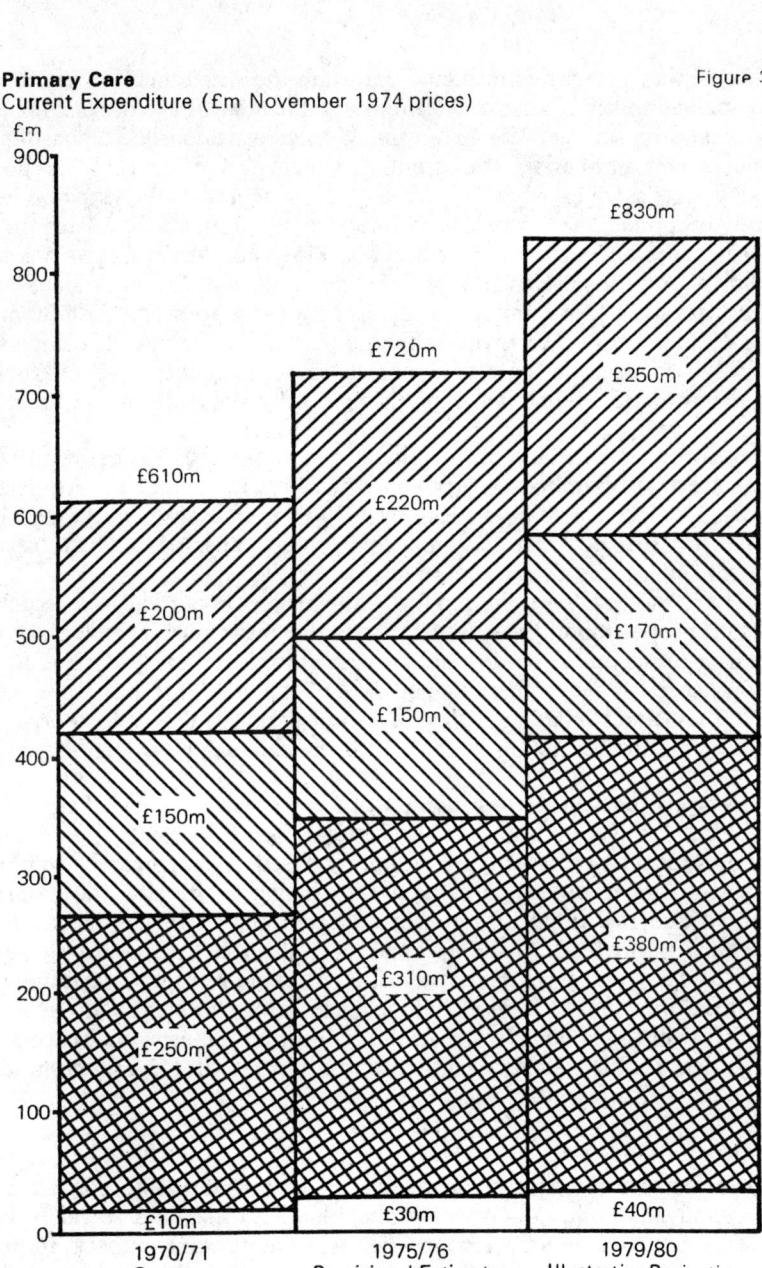

Primary Care
Current Expenditure (£m November 1974 prices)

Figure 3

£m

- £830m
- £250m
- £720m
- £220m
- £250m
- £610m
- £200m
- £170m
- £150m
- £150m
- £380m
- £310m
- £250m
- £10m
- £30m
- £40m

| 1970/71 Outturn | 1975/76 Provisional Estimate | 1979/80 Illustrative Projection |

Figures rounded to the nearest £10m. Discrepancies due to rounding

General Medical Services

General Dental and General Ophthalmic Services

Pharmaceutical Services

Health Centres, Prevention and Family Planning

21

The ideas behind preventive medicine permeate the whole field of health care from the prevention of disease and disability in the newborn to the maintenance of good health in old age. The Government have just published a consultative document which emphasises the extent to which prevention is "Everybody's Business"*. It describes what has already been achieved and explains what more can be done. The document is intended to promote discussion in the health, education and social services and encourage authorities to give a greater emphasis to preventive activities both in planning and in the allocation of resources. But even more important is to bring home to everyone how much they can do to improve their own health and that of their family. The document will be followed over the next few years by a series of papers on particular aspects of prevention which will explain more fully what action can be taken.

3.24 Preventive medicine and health education are particularly important when resources are tightly limited as they can often lead to savings in resources in other areas. An increase of about £2m by 1979/80 is envisaged for these specific preventive services. But it is also implicit in many other parts of the general strategy set out in this document. In particular the growth envisaged for the primary care services as a whole, and for health visitors in particular, who devote a significant proportion of their time to preventive measures for families, should enable more resources to be devoted to prevention. The same applies to the domiciliary social services where a good deal of the work also has a preventive aspect. In these and similar ways the Government believe that, over a period of years, the role of prevention in health and social care can be strengthened.

3.25 We suggest that authorities should at the very least maintain their present levels of health education and other activities designed to bring home to their communities the many serious types of illness caused, for example, by smoking, eating or drinking to excess. In some areas existing health education work is very limited and the authorities concerned are asked to review the need for greater effort in this field. At the national level, the Health Education Council continues to carry out general campaigns, to promote research and training in health education, and to advise and produce information and materials in support of campaigns locally by health education officers and others. In planning their health education activities, authorities should not hesitate to seek the Council's advice.

Environmental health

3.26 There are some important preventive activities—normally referred to as environmental health work—for which health authorities and social services departments are not directly responsible. Any substantial cutback in these local authority services would expose people to risk and have adverse repercussions on the NHS. For example, the food hygiene services of local authorities help to save NHS expenditure on hospital beds and drugs for food poisoning. Similarly, the effective control of epidemics of notifiable disease is essential to the NHS. The Government are hoping during the coming year to provide a new communicable disease surveillance unit under the auspices of the Public Health Laboratory Service. This will provide central support and advice to the local services when a serious outbreak of infectious disease occurs.

---

* "Prevention and Health—Everybody's Business" HMSO, price 50p.

THE GENERAL AND ACUTE HOSPITAL SERVICES AND THE MATERNITY SERVICES

The level of growth envisaged for general and acute hospital services (1·2 per cent a year) is considerably less than they have had in recent years. It would cover the burden on them of an increasing elderly population and allow for some spread of new methods of treatment. It would not permit the degree of improvement needed to meet all the pressures facing the services, particularly the need to reduce waiting times and to promote new developments. A critical scrutiny of the use of resources in these services is suggested with a view to releasing resources for further development of the acute services, and to allow for developments in other hospital services, notably geriatric medicine and mental illness. It is hoped that the professions will continue to examine the implications of different types of treatment for resource use.

Despite the sharp fall in the number of births in recent years, the cost of hospital maternity provision has considerably increased. A stringent review of maternity services is therefore suggested, with a view to reducing their cost by about 2 per cent a year.

4.1 This section is concerned primarily with the general and acute hospital services and the maternity services—including all hospital services except those concerned with geriatric medicine, mental handicap, mental illness and units for the younger disabled, which are covered in the appropriate client group sections. The general and acute hospital services draw patients from all sectors of the community, and all client groups, but the elderly in particular are important users of them.

4.2 The acute and maternity services must be planned in co-ordination with other hospital services. The pattern of hospital services recommended in the Department's circular of March 1975, DS 85/75, is based on the trend towards the greater interdependence of the various branches of medicine and the growing need to bring together a wide range of facilities for diagnosis and treatment. It includes:—

  (i) a *district general hospital* (DGH)—providing for the whole population of its district a full range of specialised treatment, and including a maternity unit, a psychiatric unit, a geriatric unit containing at least half the district geriatric beds, and a children's department, as well as specialised surgical and medical facilities. Some, but not all, DGHs would have accident and emergency units, and some would have in-patient units for ENT and ophthalmology. Some would also provide regional specialties (such as neurosurgery).

  (ii) *Community Hospitals*—for those patients not requiring the full specialist facilities of a DGH, and often nearer their homes. While arrangements will vary according to local conditions (including population density), up to a quarter of all in-patient beds and many day places might eventually be in community hospitals. It is intended that up to two-thirds of community hospital beds should be for geriatric patients and for elderly patients with severe dementia. The remainder would be medical or post-operative surgical patients including pre-convalescent cases transferred from the DGH.

4.3 The main hospital services for a district need to operate as an integrated unit. Though it may not be essential in every district, there are great advantages in providing these services on a single site. In view of the lower level of capital expenditure now proposed, it will be several decades before this can be achieved all over the country. Meanwhile, in many districts, hospital services which are together equivalent to a DGH must continue to be provided in buildings on separate sites. Where this is likely to continue for some time, health authorities have been asked to examine the possibilities of redeploying services in order to achieve wholly, or as far as possible, the implicit objectives of a DGH. The closest local co-operation is necessary to run a successful service on this basis.

4.4 Where gaps in the service are so large that some completely new building is the only answer, the *nucleus hospital* provides a possible solution. The Department is developing a design for a small hospital of about 300 beds, which would not be rigidly standard, at a basic works cost of less than £6m (at current price levels). It will provide a range of standard departments which can be selected to suit local needs. It will be viable in itself as a first phase and will be capable of expansion later on from the original nucleus to a hospital in the range of, say, 600 to 900 beds. The utmost economy in capital and running costs, consistent with maintaining acceptable medical and nursing standards, will be sought in developing the design.

4.5 Community hospitals can in many cases be created by adaptation of existing small hospitals at significantly lower cost than DGH development. The development of community hospitals will be essential to achieve the targets suggested in Sections V and VIII for geriatric provision and provision for elderly patients with severe dementia. By including in them some general medical and pre-convalescent beds it should be possible to reduce pressures on DGHs and create a more balanced range of patients and services more likely to attract staff. We suggest that authorities should do all they can to include the development of community hospitals in their plans—particularly by adaptation.

The general and acute hospital services

4.6 Current expenditure on acute in-patients and out-patients is estimated to have been about £1,220m in 1975/76; capital expenditure (including maternity services) was about £230m.

4.7 In the acute services, developments in recent years have included:—

- an increasing emphasis on shorter in-patient stay, the early ambulation of patients, and day care;
- advances in medical and scientific techniques, leading to a marked increase of demand for both capital and current resources;
- increasing awareness of the importance of rehabilitation.

4.8 There has been a considerable increase in the use of most of the services as measured by the number of patients who have been treated. Between 1970 and 1973* in-patient cases in acute specialties rose by an average of 1·1 per cent a year and out-patient attendances by 1·9 per cent a year—an increase in use

---

* Note: 1973/74 is the latest year for which both appropriately categorised financial information and matching activity statistics are available.

24

considerably larger than the increase in the population as a whole (0·3 per cent a year).

4.9 During the same period there was also:—

- an increase in the cost of the acute services by an average of 3 per cent a year at constant prices, reflecting a similar increase in overall staff numbers;
- a decrease in the number of in-patient beds by about 0·7 per cent a year;
- a decrease in the average length of in-patient stay by 2·6 per cent a year;
- an increase in the average cost of treatment per in-patient of about 2 per cent a year.

A graph showing these trends is at Figure 4.

4.10 The general trends therefore are for acute treatment to be given to more patients each year, who stay a shorter time in hospital. Treatment facilities are being used more intensively, and the total cost has been rising faster than the number of patients treated. The increase in the average cost per case is probably due to a number of factors, which it is not possible to separate. But they are likely to include the higher cost of some new forms of treatment and the greater nursing dependency of the increasing number of elderly patients.

Needs and priorities
4.11 For the acute services, as for other sectors, there are only inadequate objective indicators of the extent of current need. The increased numbers of elderly (who in 1972 accounted for 37 per cent of acute in-patients) will increase the demand for acute services, particularly in the specialty of orthopaedics, as well as for geriatric provision. Existing services differ widely between localities, but the full benefits of advances in medicine are not everywhere available to patients and the staff who treat them. For some types of treatment (for example of chronic joint disease) and diagnostic techniques (for example scanning) there has been considerable pressure to expand, but the extent of expansion has varied widely between districts. Facilities for the assessment and special care of the new born, and of very young children, are also unevenly distributed. In view of their importance for patients, these and other comparable advances represent essential growth points, which should not be neglected in localities where development is needed even during periods of severe restraint. Of no less importance is the need to improve rehabilitation services in view of their major economic and social benefits both to individuals and to the community.

4.12 Waiting times for out-patient appointments and in-patient admission, especially in the surgical specialties, provide clear evidence of inadequate provision of services. Over the past 10 years the total in-patient waiting list in England has hovered about the half-million mark, with little change from year to year. Between 1969 and 1972 there was a small and hopeful downward trend but this has now been reversed during the recent industrial unrest in the service. Waiting time is a better indicator. It would be wasteful to attempt to provide enough resources to meet *any* peak in demand. But waiting times are often unacceptably long and the recent industrial troubles have tended to make them worse.

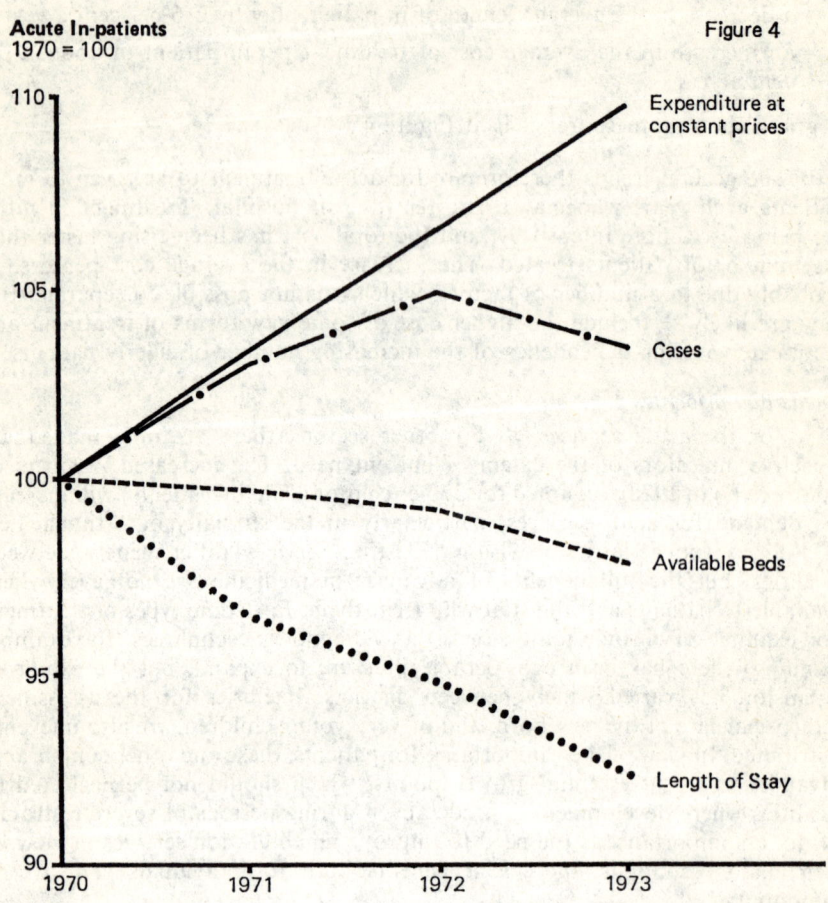

Acute In-patients
1970 = 100

Figure 4

Expenditure at constant prices

Cases

Available Beds

Length of Stay

110

105

100

95

90

1970   1971   1972   1973

The fall in the number of acute cases in 1973 may have been influenced by industrial action in that year.

Problems for resolution

4.13 The main needs, therefore, in the acute services are:—

– to reduce waiting times;

– to reduce geographical disparity, both between and within regions;

– to facilitate medical advances and improved patterns of care;

– to provide for the increased number of elderly;

– to make further improvements in the rehabilitation services.

4.14 On waiting times, the Department last year issued a circular asking authorities to review the management of their waiting lists, with the initial aim, where it has not already been achieved or bettered, of admitting all urgent cases in less than a month and all other waiting list patients in less than a year. These targets are a long way from being achieved. The circular drew attention to various types of management action that can be taken to improve the position, including increased emphasis on day surgery and the reallocation (perhaps temporarily) of resources to situations of particular need. It also asked that where the targets could not be achieved because of a shortage of resources the latter should be assessed and reported together with an estimate of the cost and practicability of overcoming it. A sum of £5m has been specially earmarked from the capital allocation for 1975/76 and subsequent years for small capital schemes which will help to reduce waiting lists.

4.15 The Resource Allocation Working Party (already referred to in Section I) has recommended that allocations to regions should aim progressively to reduce disparities between them. The Working Party's recommendations have already influenced the allocations for 1976/77, and it is now studying the problems of resource distribution within regions. Those regions which gain extra resources from this policy should be able to achieve an above average improvement of their services; those whose allocations are restricted will need to scrutinise all their services with particular care, especially the relatively expensive ones such as the specialist hospital services.

Resources to 1979/80

4.16 The central proposal in this document is that much of the available "growth money" should be concentrated on the services used mainly by the elderly and the physically handicapped, the mentally ill and handicapped, and children. The rates of growth suggested for these services would leave some scope for increasing the resources used in the acute services, but in proportionate terms the growth would be smaller—an annual average growth in current expenditure of about 1·2 per cent (including an extra allowance which has been made to take account of the phasing out of pay-beds from NHS hospitals and their use for NHS purposes). This level of growth is considerably less than these services have enjoyed in past years. But it would enable provision to be made for the increasing number of elderly in the population, and to finance some limited advances in medical techniques and improvements in patterns of care.

4.17 But it will not of itself allow the acute services to make all the improvements in services which are desirable, or to meet all the pressures in many localities. It is therefore suggested that there should be a particularly searching examination of the use of resources in these services, with the aim of releasing

27

resources for development within the acute services themselves, and for other hospital services, particularly geriatric medicine and mental illness.

Scope for rationalisation in the acute sector

4.18 During the last decade the introduction and development of the type of medical organisation discussed in the reports of the Joint Working Party on Organisation of Medical Work in Hospitals (Cogwheel), combined with changes in professional practice, have encouraged more economical and efficient patterns in the delivery of care. Lengths of stay have steadily declined and day care has been replacing in-patient care for certain procedures. These developments have released resources which, when combined with the growth in expenditure, have enabled the services to develop and expand.

4.19 There has also been a mounting volume of professional literature on such questions as out-patient/day surgery in a number of clinical conditions, the use or abuse of diagnostic tests, and methods of control of pharmaceutical expenditure in the hospital services. This reflects the growing concern of many clinicians to find new ways of combining a high quality of care with efficient use of resources. Certain operations (such as tonsillectomy and adenoidectomy and the traditional surgical treatment of haemorrhoids) are also being used more selectively. The general concern about the cost implications of different forms of treatment was illustrated in the symposium held in Winchester in 1974[1] at which clinicians from a number of fields reviewed the possibilities of increasing cost-effectiveness. Some clinicians have themselves been reassessing demands for investigations in pathology and radiology; and the Royal College of Radiologists has set up a working party to examine the over-use of radiology. An illustrative list of published reports on innovations in clinical practice is at Appendix A to this section. These suggest the possible scope for a reduction in resources used on in-patient services, without a reduction in effectiveness.

4.20 Decisions on clinical practice concerning individual patients are and must continue to be the responsibility of the clinicians concerned. But it is hoped that this document will encourage further scrutiny by the professions of the resources used by different treatment regimes. There will also need to be close scrutiny of the cost of administering the hospital services.

Use of beds

4.21 An important part of the suggested strategy will be to identify those areas and specialties which have more acute beds than are needed to provide efficient services, with particular attention to areas and specialties where provision is markedly above national averages. Some units can be closed without replacement of the services they provide, or their function can be changed either to treat the same number of patients less expensively (eg in day surgery units or in five day wards where practicable), or to provide services for the elderly or mentally ill. Views are sought on the extent to which this can be done without detriment to the overall effectiveness of medical care. Ministers recognise that this policy will, in the short term, adversely affect the convenience of some patients and their relatives and may therefore be unwelcome locally. But they hope that Community Health Councils after considering this document will support authorities where closures or changes of use can lead to greater

---

[1] The results were published in the British Medical Journal on 2, 9 and 26 November 1974.

efficiency and a better use of resources. Ministers have already made it clear that where health authorities and CHCs agree they will allow closures to go ahead without reference to them. Local protests will only be given serious consideration if they are accompanied by realistic alternative solutions within the expenditure limits.

4.22 The extent to which beds can be reduced depends significantly on the average length of in-patient stay. Within the national average for acute (Type 1) hospitals (9·8 days in 1972/73) there was a wide range between different areas, from 14·7 days in the area with the longest average stay to 6·7 days in the area with the shortest. If the average length of stay could be reduced to the present median in areas where it is above it, there would be a potential annual saving of the order of £26m in "hotel" costs. If reduction could be made to the present lower quartile the potential annual saving would be about £40m— ie an amount equivalent to an increase in the present current expenditure on acute services of about 2½ per cent. If these savings are made, the resources will become available for use in other hospital services, or for the development of the acute services themselves. The savings will of course be dependent on reducing the number of beds; otherwise expenditure will increase with increased turnover.

4.23 The Government intend to introduce legislation for the separation of private beds and facilities from NHS hospitals. One consequence of this legislation will be to release accommodation and services for general NHS use. As indicated in paragraph 4.16, an extra allowance has been made to take account of this phasing out of private beds and facilities and their use for NHS purposes.

Maternity services

4.24 Hospital maternity services are provided through consultant units in district general hospitals, and in general practitioners' maternity units. There has been a sharp fall in the number of births for several years, but the cost of hospital maternity services has considerably increased. Between 1970 and 1973, the total number of births fell by 5·0 per cent a year, the number of in-patient cases fell by an average of 1·6 per cent a year and the number of out-patient attendances by 2·6 per cent a year. The number of beds fell marginally. The average length of in-patient stay also decreased from 7·3 days to 6·9 days. Nevertheless, the cost of the service has risen by about 4 per cent a year and staff numbers have increased proportionately. An increased proportion of births has been taking place in hospital (as recommended in the Peel Report) and ante-natal care has expanded. The average cost per case rose by about 6 per cent a year in real terms. The bed occupancy rate fell from an average of 72 per cent in 1970 to 65 per cent in 1973.

A graph illustrating these trends is at Figure 5.

4.25 Though local circumstances vary considerably, we suggest that in general the hospital maternity services have attracted too large a share of resources; and that the minimum aim should be to have lowered their cost by about 7 per cent by 1979/80 (ie an annual average decrease of somewhat under 2 per cent), or about £10m for the country as a whole.

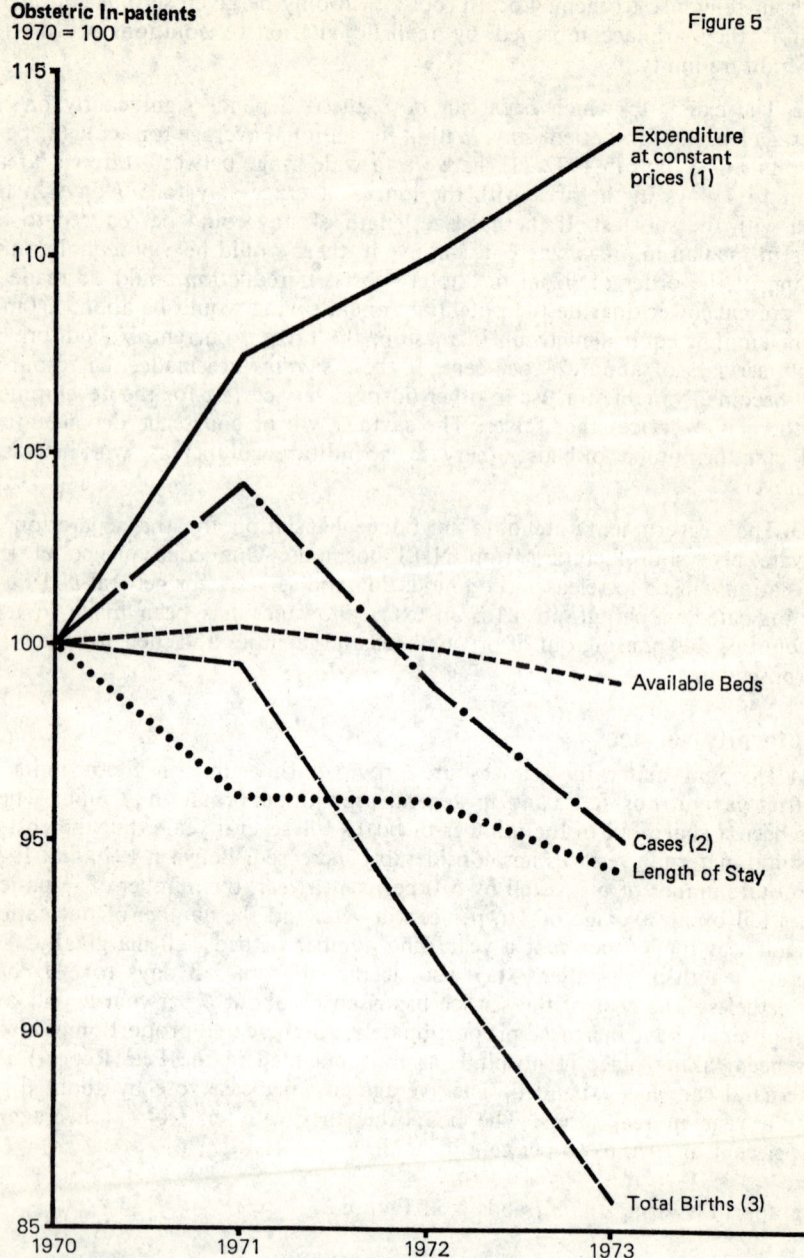

Obstetric In-patients
1970 = 100

Figure 5

115 —

Expenditure
at constant
prices (1)

110 —

105 —

100 —

Available Beds

95 —

Cases (2)

Length of Stay

90 —

85 —

1970   1971   1972   1973

Total Births (3)

(1) Estimate based on type II maternity hospitals
(2) Some 80% of cases are births
(3) Including non-hospital births

30

4.26 The "central projection" of the Office of Population Censuses and Surveys is that the number of births will start to increase in 1977, and that the increase will continue for at least 10 years. Forecasting the birthrate is widely acknowledged to be difficult, and the dilemma in present circumstances is how best to balance the need to transfer resources out of an overprovided service against a possible risk of underprovision (in particular of trained specialists) in future years.

4.27 The level of maternity services in all localities will certainly need to be stringently reviewed, and to be kept under review in the light of any local changes in the number of births. The best way of reducing provision to appropriate levels will need to be considered carefully in the light of all the existing facilities in each locality, and in consultation with the interests affected. In some there may be a case for reducing levels of provision in consultant units; in others a better course would be to make available the resources of general practitioner maternity units to other services which need them urgently. This, though naturally involving disappointment for general practitioners and those of their maternity patients who would prefer to have their babies in such units, would have the advantage of leaving intact the corpus of specialist expertise. It may be the best solution in cases where the GP unit serves a population for which there is a relatively accessible consultant department.

Transfers of acute and maternity facilities to other services

4.28 An effective scrutiny of the acute services and a reduction in expenditure on hospital maternity services should yield a substantial number of beds for use in the specialties of geriatric medicine and mental illness, both of which, as explained in the opening paragraphs of this section, are intended to have a significant proportion of their beds within district general hospitals. In addition, small hospitals can be diverted for use as community hospitals which can contribute to the care of patients who do not need the facilities of a DGH.

4.29 The measures of rationalisation suggested would benefit the geriatric and the psychiatric services, and should result in more concentrated facilities for the acute and maternity services, which should make them easier to run efficiently. The extent to which concentration is possible will vary considerably between districts; but it will be essential to make an early start on the process of rationalisation, if its benefits are to be realised.

Hospital services concerned with prevention

4.30 Those aspects of services which are particularly concerned with prevention should be given an appropriate share of growth. They include certain screening programmes, services concerned with the treatment and prevention of sexually transmitted diseases, family planning, abortion, and genetic counselling. Hospital assessment services for newly born and very young children have an important preventive role, and they too should be developed where at present they are inadequate.

Capital programme

4.31 The increase in local discretion to switch between current and capital expenditure will affect the exact size of the health capital programme, but a reduced capital programme is inevitable. A total capital expenditure on hospitals and community health of £235m in 1979/80 is projected.

4.32 A suggested division of this total between programmes is given in Table 2 of Annex 2. The proportionate share of the total devoted to mental illness and geriatrics is projected to increase, leaving £155m available for the general hospital capital programme.

4.33 It is suggested that the criteria for its use should be:—

    (i) preference for upgrading or adaptation of existing stock where possible;

    (ii) priority for capital schemes which are essential to the maintenance of the increased medical student programme;

    (iii) preference for small new developments closely related to urgent needs, particularly in deprived areas; it may be necessary to restrict major schemes (other than those in (ii) above) to those which are the only way of remedying absolute and major gaps;

    (iv) preference for projects producing greater efficiency and savings in current expenditure: small capital schemes can often assist the rationalisation of services;

    (v) concentration on economical standards of provision and design.

Conclusion

4.34 Thus it is suggested that the planning and operation of the acute and maternity services should have the following objectives:—

– to reduce long waiting times;

– to maintain development, particularly of preventive aspects of the services, services connected with rehabilitation, and general advances in medical practice and forms of care;

– to yield some resources and facilities to geriatric medicine and mental illness;

– to achieve these objectives with a lower rate of overall growth in resources than has previously been available (and with some reduction in expenditure on hospital maternity services).

4.35 This is a difficult but challenging strategy. A precondition for its success will be intensive examination of the present pattern of services and their objectives by those who provide, manage, and plan them. They will need to work in close co-operation with each other, and in close consultation with staff interests and Community Health Councils.

General and Acute Hospital and Maternity Services
Current Expenditure (£m November 1974 prices)

Figure 6

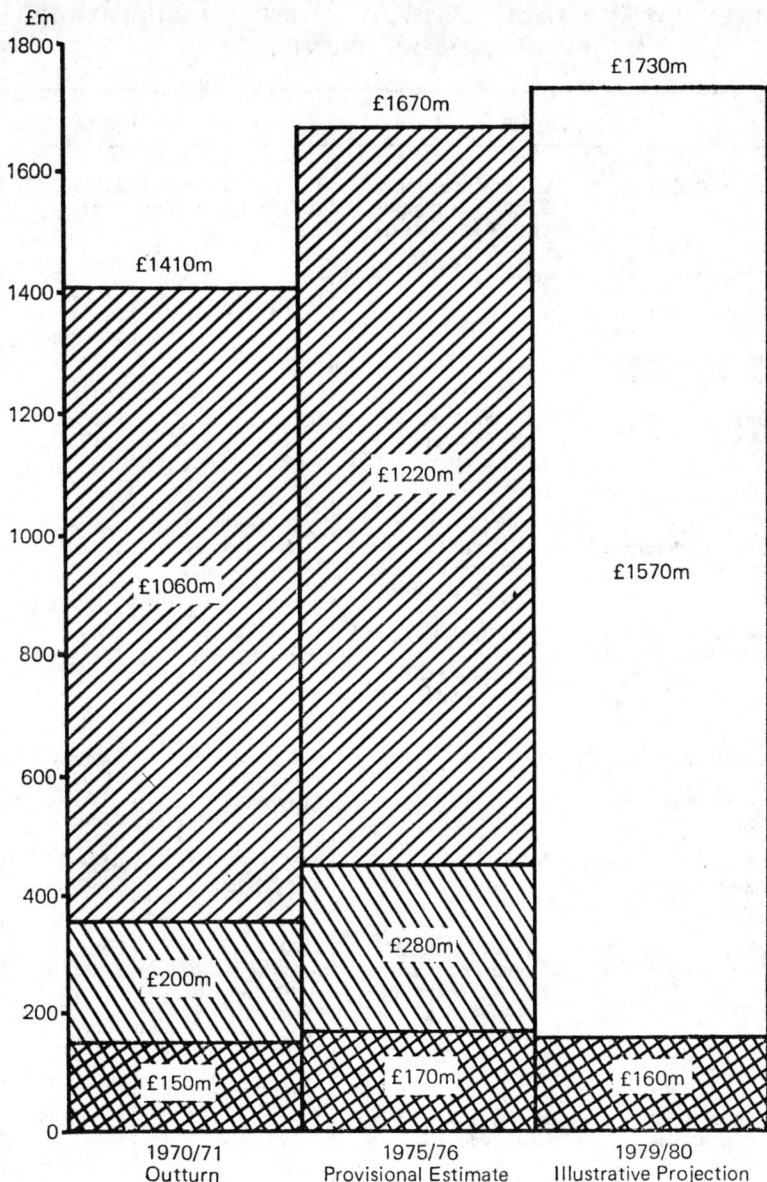

£m

£1730m

£1670m

£1410m

£1570m

£1220m

£1060m

£280m

£200m

£150m

£170m

£160m

1970/71
Outturn

1975/76
Provisional Estimate

1979/80
Illustrative Projection

Figures rounded to the nearest £10m.   This bar chart is on half scale.

Acute In-patients and Out-patients

Ambulances and Miscellaneous Hospital

Obstetric In-patients and Out-patients and Midwives

No attempt has been made to allocate expenditure between the general and acute categories in 1979/80.

ILLUSTRATIVE LIST OF PUBLISHED REPORTS ON INNOVATIONS
IN CLINICAL PRACTICE

No.	Title/Subject		Author	Publication	Year
1	Early ambulation	An early account of 485 cases of inguinal hernia treated as day patients by operation under local anaesthesia	E L Farquharson (Edinburgh)	Lancet 2, 517	1955
2	A controlled study of the effects of tonsillectomy and adenoidectomy in children		W J E McKee	Brit J Prev Soc Med	1963
3	Operating on children as day cases	The clinical management of 734 children operated upon in a 5-year period	R Lawrie (The Evelina Patty London)	Lancet 2, 1289	1964
4	Hospital stay of patients undergoing minor surgical procedures	Length of stay in hospital for patients undergoing minor surgical procedures	C R Campbell H A F Dudley (Aberdeen)	Lancet 2, 403	1964
5	A co-operative effort to remove a waiting list	The early discharge of 143 hernia patients in co-operation with district nursing and GP services	L W Aldridge (Birmingham)	BMJ 1, 183	1965
6	A controlled study evaluation of adeno-tonsillectomy in children		S R Mawson P Adlington M Evans	J Laryng 81, 777	1967
7	Rationalising requests for x-ray films in neurology		J W D Bull K J Zilkha	BMJ 4, 569-570	1968
8	Early discharge after hernia repair	A controlled trial comparing the results of 1 and 6 days' stay in hospital after operation for the repair of inguinal hernia	D Morris A W M Ward A J Handyside (Sheffield)	Lancet 1, 681	1968
9	Treatment of haemorrhoids	An out-patient technique	P Lord	Proc Roy Soc 1, 68 p. 935	1968
10	The treatment of varicose veins by injection sclerotherapy		R G Reid N G Rothnie	Brit J Surg 55 No 12	1968
	Cost of treating varicose veins	Compares in-patient surgical treatment and out-patient sclerotherapy, includes estimates of costs of NHS treatment and loss of earnings	D Piachaud J N Weddell	Lancet Vol 12, 72 p 1191	1972

No.	Title/Subject		Author	Publication	Year
11	Out-patient operations as the GP sees it	Arrangements for aftercare in the community and criteria for the selection of patients	Deen and Wilkinson	BMJ 18. 1	1969
12	Short stay surgery	Short stay and day surgery for the treatment of hernias, varicose veins and haemorrhoids	R Peatfield (Bedford)	Health Trends 1, No 2	1969
13	Out-patient operations	An analysis of surgical procedure conducted in an out-patient clinic and of intermediate surgery performed with full operating facilities on a day basis	J A Williams (Birmingham)	BMJ 1, 174	1969
14	Use of day beds in gynaecology	An account of 3,000 minor gynaecological cases treated as day patients	G A Craig (Bradford)	BMJ 2, 786	1970
15	Minor gynaecological out-patient operations	Anaesthetic techniques and the results in 143 cases are described	H Wagman D S Bamford (The London Hospital)	BMJ 20 Feb	1971
16	Day surgery	Day surgery in an autonomous unit. Arrangements for day patients requiring plastic surgery and for patients in other surgical specialties	J Calnan P Martin (Hammersmith)	BMJ 4, 92	1971
17	How much clinical investigation?	Variations in the intensity of radiological and pathological investigation in different regional hospital boards and 8 acute hospitals	J Ashley P Paster Beresford	Lancet April	1972
18	The scope and safety a short stay surgery	A study of 705 patients operated on for hernia or varicose veins and discharged 48 hours after operation	F S A Doran M White M Drury	Brit J Surgery May	1972
19	Economical use of hospital beds		P Bell D Shearer	Nursing Times 5 October	1972
20	A year in the life of a surgical day unit	Operations in plastic surgery, ENT, orthopaedic surgery and general surgery are discussed	T H Berrill (Coventry)	BMJ 11 Nov p 348	1972
21	Another approach to the hernia waiting list	How a backlog of hernia cases were worked off over a 3-week period	A D B Chant (Southampton)	Lancet Nov 11	1972

No.	Title/Subject		Author	Publication	Year
22	Is the Xylose test still a worthwhile investigation?		G E Sladen P J Kumar	BMJ 3, 223-225	1973
23	Major out-patient surgery	The clinical management of 300 patients with "intermediate" conditions operated on as day patients	Ruckley Maclean Ludgate Espley	Lancet 24 Nov	1973
24	Out-patient gynaecology	Techniques are described for diagnostic curettage, cryosurgery of the cervix and therapeutic abortion	R J Beard E Holt G Chamberlain (Queen Charlotte's)	Brit J Hospital Medicine April	1973
25	Manchester Royal Infirmary Programmed Investigation Unit	The planned admission and systematic investigation of medical patients within 5 days	Donald Longson B Young	BMJ 1 Dec	1973
26	Out-patient digital dilatation of anal canal and the rectum	A study of the method with particular reference to pain, and the recurrence of symptoms	J McCaffrey	Lancet 18 Jan	1975
27	"Tottering Home"	Comments on the SHHD Report "The value of the day bed unit in general hospital practice" and suggests further studies	Leading article	Lancet 21 June	1975
28	Anaesthetics in the Manchester Region	An attitude survey of anaesthetists on the content of their work	J Parkhouse	Brit J Anaesthesia 47, 607-614	1975
29	The provision of an anaesthetic service	A statistical approach in estimating the number of anaesthetists required for on-call emergency duty and in the planning of operation lists	A R C Jennings	Brit J Hosp Med April 404-413	1975
30	Screening Methods for Covert Bacteriuria in Schoolgirls	A study of different methods of testing comparing both false-positive and false-negative rates and costs	Bridget Edwards R H R White Heather Maxted I Deverill P A White	BMJ 31 May	1975
31	What is diagnostic radiology's place in medicine?		J W D Bull	BMJ 3, 394-400	1974
32	Use of intravenous urography		Kreel Elton Habershon Mason Meade	BMJ 4, 31-33	1974
33	The value of intravenous urography in investigating hypertension		Atkinson Kellett	Journal Royal Coll Physicians 8, 175-180	1974

No.	Title/Subject	Author	Publication	Year
34	Efficiency of routine screening and lateral chest radiographs in a hospital based population	Sagel Evens Forrest Bramson	New Eng Journal 291, 1001-4	1974
35	The preoperative chest X-ray	I H Kerr	Brit J of Anaesthesia 46, 558-63	1974
36	Plain skull roentgenograms in children with head trauma	Roberts Shopfner	Amer J of Roent 114, 230-40	1974
37	Intravenous urography in investigation of hypertension	Bailey Evans Fleming	Lancet 2, 57-58	1975
38	Unnecessary X-rays	W B James	BMJ 10 Jan	1970
39	Unnecessary X-rays	D F Thomas	BMJ 10 April	1971
40	REVIEW PUBLICATIONS Third report of the JWP on Organisation of Medical Work in Hospitals (Cogwheel)			1974
	Value of the Day Bed Unit in General Hospital Practice. Scottish Health Studies No 32	I W Kemp		1975
	Effectiveness and Efficiency	A L Cochrane	Rock Carling Fellowship	1971

V

SERVICES USED MAINLY BY THE ELDERLY

The growing proportion of the population aged 65 and over will place an increasing strain on most of the health and personal social services. The main objective of services for elderly people is to help them remain in the community for as long as possible. It is, however, important to provide hospital and residential care for old people unable to live independently in the community: and to improve hospital facilities for early diagnosis, intensive treatment and rehabilitation.

Subject to local circumstances, the following national targets are suggested:—

- expansion of the home nursing (and health visiting) services by 6 per cent a year, of the chiropody services by 3 per cent a year, and of home helps and the meals services by 2 per cent a year;
- an increase in the number of local authority residential places by 2,000 a year, to be concentrated where local needs are greatest, and of day centre places by 600 a year;
- an additional 1,150 hospital geriatric beds a year, and the provision of a progressively increasing proportion of geriatric beds in general hospitals;
- provision of 2,000 beds a year in community hospitals for old people, including those with severe mental infirmity, to replace provision in unsatisfactory long-stay hospitals.

Effective joint planning between local and health authorities is particularly important. The voluntary sector will continue to have a major role to play in the provision of services for the elderly.

5.1 There are now more than 6½ million people aged 65 or over in England and they comprise about 14 per cent of the total population. Since 1961 the total population has grown by 7 per cent, but the over 65s have increased by over 25 per cent. This trend will continue until 1981. By 1980 nearly 15 per cent of the population will be 65 or over. The number of over 75s, who are the heaviest users of health and personal social services, is expected to rise by half a million over ten years from 2·3 millions to 2·8 millions (from about 5 per cent to about 6 per cent of the total population).

5.2 Old people are major users of most of the health and personal social services. The primary care and acute hospital services are very important to them. But those services which are mainly or entirely used by the elderly will have to meet a particularly sharp increase in demand. Moreover, social and environmental changes such as smaller housing units and increased job mobility have tended to reduce the ability of younger people to care for the elderly in a family environment.

5.3 The general aim of policy is to help the elderly maintain independent lives in their own homes for as long as possible. The main emphasis is thus on the development of the domiciliary services and on the promotion of a more active approach towards the treatment of the elderly in hospital. But old people who can no longer continue to live independently in the community even with the support of all available health and social services will need long term residential or hospital care. This need will increase with the number of elderly and in particular with the number of people over 75.

Services used mainly by the elderly

5.4 Many of the services used by the elderly are used also by physically handicapped people in other age groups. Services (for example home nursing and residential accommodation) used mainly by the elderly are considered in this section, and those (such as aids and adaptations) used mainly by the younger physically handicapped are covered in the next section. However, the importance of many of the services to both groups should be borne in mind.

Services for the Elderly living at home

5.5 About 95 per cent of all elderly people are living in the community and family doctors meet most of their medical needs. The primary health care and community services of which the elderly are major users are listed below. Here, and in the following paragraphs on residential and hospital provision, the Departmental guidelines for standards of service are given where they exist, but they are under review.

Home Helps. In 1974 there were about 41,000 whole-time equivalent home helps, ie 6 per 1,000 elderly. The guideline is for a ratio of 12 per 1,000.

Meals. About 600,000 meals are served each week through the meals-on-wheels services and day centres and clubs. The guideline is for 200 per week per 1,000 elderly—about 1,300,000 overall.

Home Nursing. Over half the time of home nurses is thought to be spent on the elderly. In 1974 there were about 11,000 home nurses in all—somewhat less than 1 per 4,000 total population. The guideline is for 1 per 2,500–4,000 according to local needs.

Day centres. In 1974 there were about 23,000 day centre places available to the elderly and the younger physically handicapped. About half of these are used by elderly people, giving about 2 places per 1,000 elderly. The guideline is 3-4 places per 1,000.

Chiropody. Chiropody services do a great deal to prevent immobility, and nearly all of them are delivered to the elderly. In 1974 there were about 1,400 whole-time equivalent chiropodists (about 1 per 5,000 elderly).

In addition, social workers help old people, and housing conditions are a key influence on the ability of old people to continue to manage in the community and on the quality of their lives. Voluntary effort also plays an important part in meeting the needs of the elderly.

Residential Facilities

5.6 In 1974 there were about 125,000 local authority places available for elderly people and for the younger physically handicapped and others, including places supported by local authorities in voluntary or private homes. Of these, about 120,000 were provided in homes for old people, ie about 18·5 places per 1,000 elderly. The guideline is 25 places per 1,000 elderly.

Hospital Facilities

5.7 Excluding maternity and psychiatry, over 50 per cent of all hospital beds are used by people aged 65 and over. A high proportion of surgical beds is occupied by elderly people, although normally none are specifically set aside for them. For medical conditions, old people are admitted to general medical beds, or to beds designated for geriatric medicine. The factors determining whether admission is to a geriatric bed or a general medical bed vary considerably from one area to another and depend on local practice as well as available facilities. At 31 December 1974 there were 8·57 beds per 1,000 elderly specifically designated as "geriatric"; the guideline is 10 per 1,000. The present statistical separation of most geriatric services from "acute" services has contributed to the widespread belief that geriatric services are primarily concerned with providing long stay back-up facilities for the acute services. This belief is misplaced. It is estimated that over 80 per cent of patients admitted to geriatric beds remain there for less than three months. A modern geriatric service needs to provide for the direct admission of acutely medically ill elderly patients and in this aspect of its service does not differ from other acute specialities. It therefore requires equivalent facilities. Most geriatric departments now include day hospitals and out-patient clinics as well as in-patient facilities.

Elderly People with Mental Infirmity

5.8 It is estimated that about 16,000 elderly people with severe mental infirmity are in long-stay mental illness hospitals—about 2·5 per 1,000 elderly. The guidelines are 2·5 to 3 beds in local hospital units and 2 to 3 day hospital places per 1,000 elderly. There is also a larger number (one estimate puts them at well over 650,000) with varying degrees of mental infirmity associated with old age living at home or with relatives, or in various types of local authority, voluntary, and private residential accommodation.

The general picture

5.9 As stated, the Department's guidelines are under review, but the extent to which services at present fall short of them suggests a serious need for improvement.

5.10 Further, the pattern of provision often prevents help being given to those most in need with the result that residential and hospital facilities are not put to the best use. Inadequate domiciliary services cause misuse of hospital beds and unnecessary demand for residential places. Most local authorities have waiting lists for admission to residential homes, and in many instances can admit only emergency cases. Health authorities find that hospital beds are blocked by patients who could be discharged if domiciliary or residential care, or suitable housing, were available. As a consequence, other patients cannot be offered the prompt hospital treatment and rehabilitation which could lead to their own early return home.

Priorities and resources

5.11 Helping old people to remain in the community for as long as possible will require an expansion in all sectors of care, including provision of suitable housing and encouragement of greater activity by the elderly, where possible by continuing employment. The Department is currently reviewing the spectrum of services for the elderly. Research is being sponsored to get information which will be used in the review of current guidelines. High priority is being given to examining ways of making better use of hospital provision. This includes examination of the relationship between general and geriatric medicine, and the interface between geriatric medicine and other specialities. It is hoped that this will allow a more definitive formulation of the scope and scale of geriatric services for the future. As regards housing the Department of the Environment will shortly be consulting local authority associations and the main voluntary bodies concerned about the content of an up-to-date circular on housing for old people.

5.12 It is clear that even with present constraints on the HPSS as a whole there must be growth of services for the elderly, in order to keep up with their increasing number and to develop the emphasis on community care. We therefore suggest that between 1975/76 and 1979/80 current expenditure on these services should increase by about 3 per cent a year from about £550m in 1975/76 to £620m in 1979/80, and that they should benefit from a considerable proportion of available capital.

5.13 If the best use is to be made of this increase, careful thought will need to be given in each locality to the most effective patterns of development. It is suggested that, unless local needs clearly dictate a different order of priorities, particular attention should be paid to:—

- the rapid development of health and social service domiciliary services—notably home nursing (and health visiting), but also the meals and home help services and general social work support;

- the development of acute geriatric units in general hospitals with immediate access to full diagnostic, therapeutic and rehabilitation facilities, and the replacement as fast as possible of old long-stay geriatric hospitals by provision in community hospitals. Where, however, it remains necessary to keep the old long-stay hospitals, some upgrading and improvement should be undertaken to make a tolerable environment;

- the development of local authority residential homes, in the light of local circumstances;

- the development of special in-patient and day hospital units for the elderly severely mentally infirm in community hospitals as part of the district psychiatric service.

5.14 However, it should be emphasised that for the elderly co-ordinated planning is required across administrative boundaries. Joint Consultative Committees and Joint Care Planning Teams should be fully used to co-ordinate planning between the health and the personal social services, but co-ordination of the latter with other local authority services is equally important. As stated, housing is of special importance to the elderly and every effort should be made to increase the amount of sheltered housing. The Housing Act 1974 facilitates this, and housing associations should be encouraged to exploit its provisions as fully as possible.

Domiciliary Services
5.15 The more these can be expanded, the more the pressure on residential accommodation and on hospitals can be eased. On a national basis, we suggest that expenditure on *home nursing* (and *health visiting*) should be increased by 6 per cent a year, and that *chiropody services* should also be increased—we suggest by 3 per cent a year. For *home helps* and *meals* a smaller increase will be necessary because of other pressures on the personal social services. We suggest 2 per cent a year.

41

5.16 Some of these suggested growth rates exceed the annual increase in the elderly population, and should therefore permit some improvement in the standard and scope of provision and help to keep to a minimum the use of residential accommodation which is expensive in both capital and staff. The level of provision of domiciliary services varies very considerably between localities. In some (including some localities where there is a high proportion of retired people) there is a very serious lack of these services. We suggest that in these localities an especially high priority should be given to building up domiciliary care.

5.17 Within the suggested allocation of resources to the elderly, it is not possible to give the degree of protection suggested for current expenditure and at the same time maintain the *day centre capital programme* at its present level. On current average costs per place it would not be possible to maintain a day centre building programme of more than 600 places a year for the elderly and physically handicapped, but a larger programme would be possible if the average cost per place could be reduced by providing more modest facilities, perhaps using adapted buildings. Encouragement might also be given to the voluntary sector to maintain and expand its contribution in this field.

Residential Care

5.18 The pattern of provision varies considerably between localities. Two important factors which influence the amount of residential accommodation needed are the local social structure and the physical environment. In general a greater need for residential accommodation is likely in those localities with a large number of old people living alone in unsatisfactory accommodation, remote from relatives, friends, shops and other facilities. Such need may arise particularly in retirement areas. Provision of sheltered housing may reduce this need, provided the local allocation procedures are suitable.

5.19 But there will still be many old people for whom there is no alternative to residential care. The judgement of how much more residential provision is needed on a national scale is inevitably very difficult. If the stock of residential places were to keep pace with the increased number of over 75s (who take up about three-quarters of the present number of places), without allowing for any replacement of unsatisfactory ex-workhouse or other adapted premises, an annual increase of 2,500 or more places for the elderly would be necessary. However, in view of the difficulty of the judgement on a national scale and the expense of these facilities in relation to the domiciliary services, we suggest that over the next three or four years of severe economic constraint a particularly close examination of needs in each locality should be made, and that a slightly lower rate of increase—2,000 a year—may have to be aimed at. It is hoped that authorities will continue to use the facilities for the residential care of elderly people provided in homes run by voluntary bodies.

Hospitals

Acute Geriatric Provision

5.20 Few areas have enough geriatric beds in general hospitals with immediate access to diagnostic, therapeutic and rehabilitation facilities, and with provision for old people presenting as acute medical emergencies to be directly admitted under the care of the geriatric physician. There is mounting evidence that the existence of an acute geriatric service on these lines not only increases turnover, reduces waiting lists and lessens the demand for long-stay care by preventing irreversible deterioration, but also helps to prevent blocking of other beds— particularly general medical, general surgical and orthopaedic. The presence of acute geriatric beds in a general hospital enhances liaison between geriatric medicine and the other specialties which in itself contributes to better use of available resources.

5.21 It has for some years been departmental policy—supported by many professional interests—that at least 50 per cent of geriatric beds should be in general hospitals, but progress has been disappointing. Nearly one-fifth of all health districts have no geriatric beds in general hospitals. We consider that the achievement of a considerably faster rate of growth of geriatric provision in general hospitals should be accepted by health authorities as a major priority in the coming years and propose to issue detailed guidance on this in due course.

5.22 The progress should be achieved by a combination of new building and the change of use of existing beds. Provision of about 1,150 additional geriatric beds a year will be necessary to keep pace with the increasing number of elderly. The aim should be to site these additional beds in general hospitals. As suggested in Section IV, there should be considerable scope in the coming years for converting general medical and surgical beds into geriatric beds, and the NHS private beds which become available to NHS patients from the programme of phasing out should increase the scope for such transfers. Some of the private beds themselves might be suitable, but whether or not the actual beds are so converted we suggest that authorities should ensure that increases in their NHS bed stock from private beds should be wholly or largely used for the benefit of the geriatric sector.

5.23 Interim targets are proposed to secure more rapid progress towards a satisfactory pattern of geriatric provision. In all districts a minimum of 10 per cent of geriatric bed need, or one geriatric ward, whichever is the greater, should be provided in general hospitals by the end of 1976/77. There should follow a continuous programme of expansion designed to bring the level up to at least 30 per cent by the end of 1979/80. This is an interim minimum target for all health authorities; as soon as it is achieved in a particular district, the authority should proceed to the full 50 per cent target as fast as possible. Authorities are asked to give early consideration to means by which the desired change in the structure of their geriatric provision can be achieved. The Department proposes to ask authorities to submit outline proposals for meeting the interim targets. Consideration will be given to the desirability of making a central allocation of funds specifically for schemes designed to increase acute geriatric provision if that appears to be the only method of ensuring the necessary progress.

5.24 *Day hospitals* are important in a modern geriatric service, and an annual increase of 500 places in general hospitals and a further 500 in community hospitals is suggested.

Other Geriatric Provision

5.25 The standard of accommodation and overcrowding in some existing geriatric units is unacceptable even with the present limitation of resources. We suggest that resources should be set aside to maintain a programme of improving or replacing the sub-standard provision mainly through the community hospital programme at a rate of about 1,000 beds a year. If, because of slow progress in the community hospital programme, this level of provision cannot be attained, it will be important to spend some capital on the improvement of existing long-stay geriatric units.

Health Capital

5.26 We suggest that, of the proposed geriatric capital programme of about £28m a year, some two-thirds should be for general hospital provision and one-third for community hospitals (mainly by adapting existing hospitals) and improvement of existing long-stay hospitals.

Provision for the elderly suffering from mental infirmity

5.27 It is important that the run-down of mental hospitals, which is a part of the refashioning of services for the mentally ill, should not exceed the pace at which special units can be provided in community hospitals for elderly people suffering from a severe degree of mental infirmity. Capital provision rising to £7m a year by 1979/80, representing about 1,000 beds a year, is suggested for such units in Section VIII. Regard must also be paid to the extent to which residential accommodation and other supportive and domiciliary services are available for those who suffer from lesser degrees of mental infirmity and do not require continuous hospital care.

VI

SERVICES FOR THE PHYSICALLY HANDICAPPED

The main aim of services for the physically handicapped is to enable them to lead as full and useful a life as possible by providing appropriate support services and care within the community. They will gain from the expansion of home nursing, the meals services and home help suggested in Section V.

A high rate of expansion (9 per cent a year) is suggested for home aids and adaptations and certain other services provided under Section 2 of the Chronically Sick and Disabled Persons Act 1970 which make an important contribution to the mobility and quality of life of the physically handicapped.

Further local community day centre places should be provided. Attention should be paid to the needs of the blind and the deaf for social work support.

On the hospital side it is suggested that special units for the disabled should have some priority claim on the reduced capital programme; that the possibility of establishing a spinal injuries unit in the South of England should be carefully considered; and that the hospital services (including preventive services) of importance to the disabled and physically handicapped should be maintained.

6.1 Services used mainly by three groups—physically handicapped of all ages, the deaf and hard of hearing, and people who are visually handicapped—are considered here. The services include social work support, aids and adaptations to help the disabled in their home and working lives, occupational therapy, local authority day centres and residential care, special hospital units for the younger disabled, special hospital units for the treatment of spinal injuries and patients with paraplegia and tetraplegia, hearing aids and other assistance to the deaf and hard of hearing, and various types of assistance to the blind and partially sighted. The only services costed separately in Annex 2 are local authority aids, adaptations and other support services (such as provision of telephones and holidays). These services started a few years ago from a negligible or non-existent base and expenditure has now grown to about £12m. Central Government also provide certain services for the disabled, notably artificial limbs and appliances and the invalid vehicles service (current annual cost £30m).

6.2 Voluntary agencies also make an important contribution to the well-being of handicapped people of all kinds.

6.3 The Government are phasing in a mobility allowance of £260 a year for children aged five and over and adults of working age who are unable or virtually unable to walk. The cost of this allowance will be met from the Department's Social Security funds, and is not therefore a charge on health or localauthority budgets—but the amount to be spent centrally on mobility for the disabled is expected to be three times greater, an increase from £13m (the vehicle scheme element in the £30m above) to £39m annually.

Size of the groups

6.4 There is a lack of reliable information on the size of the groups, but they may be roughly as follows:—

> *Physically Disabled*—There are of the order of 350,000 adults under 65 and 50,000 children living at home. In 1974 there were about 11,000 adults in local authority or local authority sponsored residential homes, about

5,000 in long-stay hospital units (including 1,000 in units for the young disabled), and about 1,500 children in long-stay hospital units.

Deaf and Hard of Hearing of all ages—Estimates suggest that about 3 per cent to 4 per cent of the total population have a hearing impairment, of whom a small minority are totally deaf.

Blind and Partially Sighted of all ages—In 1972/73 there were 97,000 registered blind in England, and 36,900 registered partially sighted, but the latter figure is substantially below the number thought to exist.

It is not possible to estimate to what extent the numbers of physically handicapped will change in the future. But the numbers of those whose hearing or sight is impaired seem likely to rise with the increasing number of elderly.

Objectives and priorities

6.5 The main objective is to enable the younger physically handicapped to lead as full and useful a life as possible, by providing appropriate support services (including support from the community nursing service) and care within the community. A proportion of the handicapped will nevertheless need treatment or care in hospital units or residential accommodation, because of the nature and severity of their handicap or because they choose to live in that way. The objective in such cases should be to provide a high standard of care coupled with an effective rehabilitation service enabling as many as possible to return to the community with minimum risk.

6.6 On the *hospital side*, the most important need is for the establishment of a spinal injuries unit in the South of England (there is at present no such unit south of Stoke Mandeville). The priority that this should be given in the capital programme will need to be carefully assessed. A second important need is for an increase in the number of special units for the younger disabled, so that they can be given the care that is suitable for their needs, and are not unsuitably accommodated with elderly people in geriatric wards. Between 1971 and 1976 a special capital allocation of £7m was made and this has made a substantial contribution to extending provision. After 1976/77 it will not be possible to continue expenditure on this scale within the reduced capital programme. Nevertheless, we suggest that these units should have some priority claim and provision for annual expenditure of about £0·5m between 1977/78 and 1979/80 would seem reasonable. We also suggest that, in the planning and management of acute hospital services special care should be taken to ensure that other hospital services of special importance to these groups (units for the treatment of spinal injuries, paraplegia and tetraplegia, and the out-patient services which particularly affect those with sight or hearing impairment) are maintained at a satisfactory level.

6.7 It has been accepted that service provision for the deaf and hard-of-hearing should be given some priority. The main objectives are to improve the standards in audiology departments and hearing-aid centres by expansion of staff and facilities, including facilities for follow-up and rehabilitation of patients provided with hearing aids. One specific objective concerns the present behind-the-ear hearing aid programme which is due to be completed by 1979/80, by which time annual central expenditure on the programme is expected to have increased from about £5m to over £8m.

Services mainly for Elderly and Physically Handicapped
Current Expenditure (£m November 1974 prices)

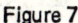
Figure 7

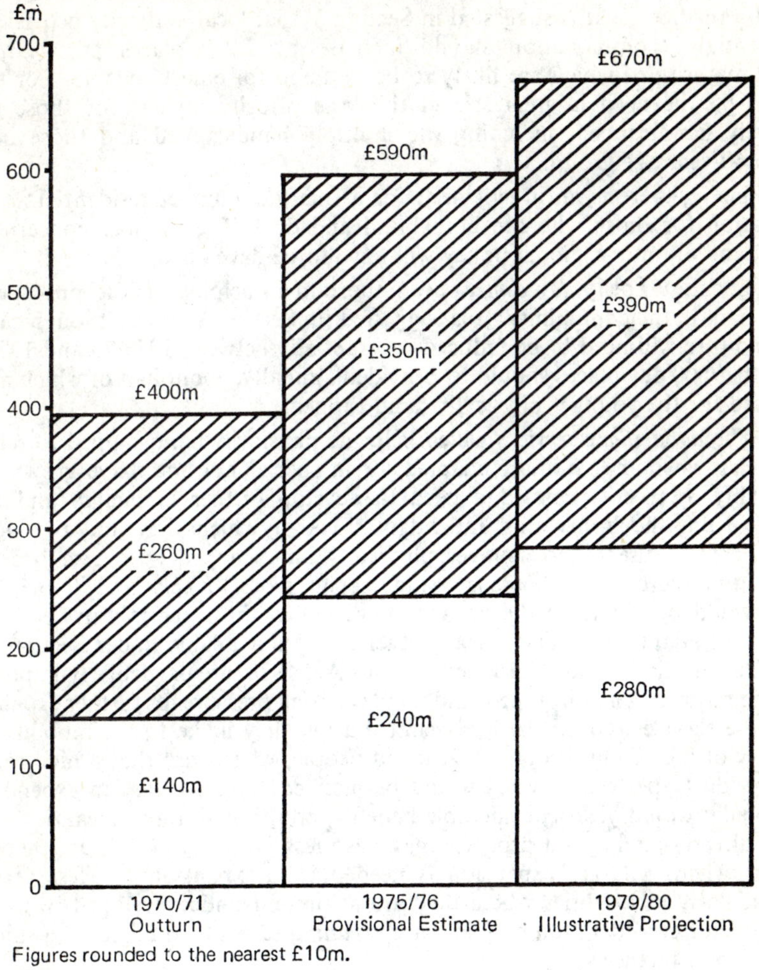

£m

700 —

£670m

£590m

600 —

£390m

500 —

£350m

£400m

400 —

£260m

300 —

200 —

£280m

£240m

100 —

£140m

0 —

| 1970/71 | 1975/76 | 1979/80 |
| Outturn | Provisional Estimate | Illustrative Projection |

Figures rounded to the nearest £10m.

Geriatric and Younger Disabled In-patients and Residential Care

Care within Community: Geriatric Out-patients
Non psychiatric Day-patients
Home Nursing
Chiropody
Home Help
Meals
Day Care
Aids, Adaptations, Phones and Holidays
Services for the Disabled

Hospital expenditure for 1975/76 and 1979/80 divided between IP and OP on
basis of same growth rates for each as for total

6.8 *Of the local authority services*, purpose-built *residential accommodation* for the younger disabled is a key provision for those who are unable to remain in their own homes but do not need to be in hospital. There are 33 residential homes provided by local authorities for this group under Part III of the National Assistance Acts, and according to latest information authorities intend to build a further 15. It is suggested in Section V that local authority provision of residential accommodation should increase by 2,000 places per year, the large majority of which are likely to be required for elderly people. For those under 65 the need is greatest and thus the priority highest for those most severely handicapped, including the multiply handicapped and those in the 40 to 60 year age group.

6.9 Finally, there is an urgent need for a small amount of residential accommodation for those who are both blind and deaf. The number concerned is small and an inter-regional policy will have to be developed.

6.10 Local authority *day centres* are important in helping handicapped people to remain in the community. It is suggested (in Section V) that although capital expenditure will need to be reduced substantially between 1975/76 and 1979/80 a further 600 day places should be provided annually, about half of which might be used for the younger physically handicapped.

6.11 The *domiciliary services* which help the physically handicapped to remain in their own homes suitably adapted, or in special housing, have grown considerably in recent years, and need to develop further in quality and type. Apart from the home aids and adaptations of which they and the elderly are the main users, the younger physically handicapped have also benefited from the increase in home nursing, social work, meals and home help, and would benefit from the growth suggested in those services in Section V. Aids and adaptations, and certain other services available under Section 2 of the Chronically Sick and Disabled Persons Act 1970, are particularly important for the physically handicapped, and there is strong pressure for further expansion of these services. Given the great contribution they make to the mobility and quality of life of physically handicapped people, we suggest that a high rate of expansion (9 per cent a year) would be justified. This increase in expenditure nationally would yield considerable benefits, and though those localities which have already made good progress may have less ground to catch up, there are others where a larger expansion is needed. The expansion of these services (particularly in localities where they are at present underdeveloped) would be suitable for consideration by joint care planning teams, and might be a suitable use of joint finance.

6.12 Social work support is a key provision for blind and partially-sighted people, and we suggest that there is considerable scope for its improvement. In particular, questions of specialist training and appropriate career opportunities for local authority staff merit concern. There is also a need to develop social service provision for deaf people.

6.13 The services covered here are for those with established handicapping conditions. Preventive measures to identify the risk of permanent handicaps in the new born and the young (for example, screening services to detect hearing impairment in young children) are vitally important if the incidence of handicap is to be reduced. The Department's consultative document on Prevention will be relevant here, as is the suggestion in Section IV that paediatric assessment units should be provided where at the moment they are lacking.

VII

SERVICES FOR THE MENTALLY HANDICAPPED

The long-term aims for these services remain those proposed in the White Paper "Better Services for the Mentally Handicapped" (Cmnd 4683): the provision of a satisfactory environment either at home or in residential accommodation; avoiding unnecessary segregation; developing ability by education and training, and support for families. Full implementation of the White Paper targets was envisaged as taking place over a 20-year period. The White Paper strategy should be substantially maintained. The priorities for the period to 1979/80 should, it is suggested, be:

- to maintain the target growth of local authority training centres and residential homes. For training centres a capital programme of about £6m is proposed to provide about 2,400 places annually, and for residential homes a programme of about £10m to provide 1,000 places annually.

- to improve staffing ratios and facilities in hospital services for the mentally handicapped. It is proposed that current expenditure on these services should increase by about 1·6 per cent a year, with a capital programme of about £9m a year to provide for occupation and training facilities, as well as essential maintenance and upgrading.

7.1 There are estimated to be about 110,000 severely mentally handicapped people in England, and more than 350,000 with mild mental handicap. In 1974 nearly 60,000 were in residential care—9,000 in local authority homes, 50,000 in hospitals—and over 10,000 in lodgings, foster homes, etc. The general aims of services for mentally handicapped people are to ensure that they have a satisfying environment (which should as far as possible be within the general community), and to provide education, social stimulation and purposeful occupation and employment so as to develop and exercise all the skills they can acquire.

7.2 A parallel strand of policy is prevention, by developing measures (for example control of environmental hazards, genetic counselling, ante-natal and perinatal care) to reduce both the incidence of mental handicap and its severity. The development of assessment services for handicapped children is considered in Section IX on services for children and their families (paragraph 9.6). From present knowledge it appears that prevention may reduce incidence sufficiently to cancel out the increased prevalence which would otherwise result from increasing longevity.

Long-term objectives
General
7.3 The long-term aim is to achieve the pattern of services proposed in *Better Services for the Mentally Handicapped*, viz:—

- to provide a satisfactory environment whether at home, in hospitals or residential accommodation;
- to avoid unnecessary segregation;
- to provide education, training and occupation to develop ability;
- to support families and help them to cope as long as possible.

Apart from the services specifically discussed below, various others such as social work, family doctors, home nursing, health visiting and holidays are used by the mentally handicapped according to their individual needs.

Hospital services

7.4 Hospitals for the mentally handicapped have historically been large and remote from the communities they serve—many were originally established as "colonies" with a deliberate policy of segregation from the outside community. They are often overcrowded. Their role in the new pattern of services is to provide treatment under specialist medical supervision, where appropriate on a day-patient or out-patient basis, rather than the residential care which, in the absence of alternative accommodation, they provide for many mentally handicapped patients at present. They should provide long-term residential accommodation only for mentally handicapped patients requiring constant nursing care under specialist supervision, for example because of severe physical disability or serious behaviour disorder. Hospital units should be planned to provide a local service, fully integrated with other services, with each unit as a rule serving a single district—in other words a population generally not exceeding 250,000. With the recommended ratio of 68 beds to 100,000 total population, future hospitals would not have more than, say, 200 beds. Some less dependent mentally handicapped hospital patients would be accommodated in smaller hostels, sited more within the community.

Residential homes

7.5 Residential care, for those mentally handicapped people unable, even with supporting services, to live in the family home (or in sheltered lodgings), is provided by local authorities. The White Paper emphasises that homes should be integrated as fully as possible with the local community, with residents living in small groups.

Training services

7.6 The parallel expansion of occupation and training services is given equal emphasis in the White Paper. Adult training centres play a key role in helping the mentally handicapped to develop and make the fullest use of their abilities. They provide education, training and occupation for mentally handicapped adults living either at home, in hospital, or in local authority residential accommodation. (Special schools for mentally handicapped children are provided by local education authorities.)

Progress in implementation

7.7 It was envisaged in the White Paper that the full development of the new pattern of services would take place over a period of about 20 years. The general aims of the White Paper were reaffirmed by the Government last year but it is recognised that policies need to be kept under review in the light of experience as services develop. Accordingly, a National Development Group for Mental Handicap, under the Chairmanship of Professor Mittler of the Hester Adrian Research Centre, has recently been appointed to play an active part in the development of departmental policy and the strategy for its implementation.

7.8 The aim has been to keep to the 20-year timescale suggested in the White Paper. Local authority expenditure in this period has been approximately on target, although loan sanctions for new building starts in 1974/75 fell some 25 per cent below target because of the previous Government's December 1973 expenditure cuts. In 1975/76 loan sanctions have returned to about the White Paper level. The number of places in residental homes has grown from under 6,000 in 1969 to some 9,500 in 1974. Even so local authorities can accommodate only a minority of those who would benefit from residential care. The number of places in adult training centres increased from about 23,000 in 1969 to some 32,000 in 1974 and is continuing to increase.

7.9 The initiatives taken by previous Governments, and the injection of substantial additional resources, have led to much improvement in the standards of care at hospitals and in the number of nursing staff. The reduction in the number of hospital beds, from about 60,000 in 1969 to 55,000 in 1974, represents further relief of pressure and overcrowding. Substantial amounts of capital have also been spent on improving buildings. However, there are still considerable shortcomings.

7.10 Full achievement of the White Paper proposals by the early 1990s implies that by 1985 there would need to be some 22,000 places in local authority homes compared with the 1974 figure of 9,500, and about 60,000 places in training centres compared with about 32,000 in 1974. This means an annual programme of over 1,000 residential places and about 2,400 training places, and a corresponding increase in staff numbers. At the same time the number of available hospital beds would be expected to fall from its current level of some 55,000 to around 46,000 in 1985. Any saving in hospital expenditure resulting from the reduced number of beds would be outweighed by an increase of perhaps more than 50 per cent over the period in expenditure per occupied bed. This would reflect both an improvement in the quality of care and the greater dependency of the remaining in-patient population as the more self-sufficient came increasingly to be cared for in the community. By 1985, for example, the ratio of nurses to in-patients would be expected to rise to 1:1.6 from its present level of 1:2.4. A substantial increase is also needed in facilities for treating day patients in hospital, though in absolute terms these would represent only a small share of the total resources required. Similarly a substantial increase is needed in various domiciliary services but these cannot be precisely quantified.

7.11 In summary, the White Paper targets and the progress made by 1974 towards meeting them, compared to the position in 1969, are as follow:

NUMBER OF PLACES PROVIDED IN 1969 AND 1974 AND WHITE PAPER TARGETS FOR 1991

	Provided 1969		Provided 1974		White Paper Target for 1991	
	Total	per 100,000 population	Total	per 100,000 population	Total	per 100,000 population
Residential Care Local authority, voluntary and private homes						
Adult	4,200	9	7,800	17	28,900	60
Child	1,700	4	1,800	4	4,800	10
Total	5,900	13	9,500*	21	33,700	70
Hospital						
Adult					26,500	55
Child					6,300	13
Total	60,000	131	55,000	119	32,800	68
Adult Training Centres	23,200	50	32,000	68	72,200	150

*Discrepancy due to rounding.

Suggested developments to 1979/80

7.12 Services for the mentally handicapped form the smallest of the main groups of services considered in this document and one which until recently was much neglected. It is important that the momentum of improvement gathered in the past few years should not be lost. The proposals which follow would maintain the development of local authority services in line with the White Paper time-scale and would also permit substantial progress in improving existing hospital services.

7.13 The primary aim is to ensure that mentally handicapped people are looked after in the community wherever this is most suitable; the development of services which this requires will of course indirectly help the remaining hospital patients by relieving pressure on the hospitals. It is therefore proposed that, as the first priority in the mental handicap field, the growth of local authority services should be maintained at the rates of about 2,400 *training centre places* and about 1,000 *residential places* a year required to achieve the White Paper targets by the early 1990s. This will require capital investment of about £6m a year for training centres and £10m a year for residential homes. The corresponding annual growth rates for current expenditure would be about 6·5 per cent and 7 per cent respectively. The National Development Group agree that priority for the expansion of local authority services would best serve the interests of the mentally handicapped; the development of training services which, despite rapid expansion in the past few years, are still not available for many mentally handicapped people living with their families, is particularly urgent. Within the residential programme priority should be given to enabling children to be kept out of hospital care: the number of local authority places for mentally handicapped children, though increasing, is not rising fast enough to match the undoubted priority for this category. There is also a possibility of accommodating a small number of children in the other ways, for example fostering.

7.14 Many hospitals for the mentally handicapped do not have the staff and facilities to provide an active modern service, and since the fall in the number of patients can only be very gradual the second priority in this field is to maintain real improvement in *hospital standards*—particularly where they are least satisfactory at present. The most important factor here is the level of current expenditure and it is proposed that this should increase at about 1·6 per cent annually, equivalent to a 3 per cent improvement in standards when the falling number of in-patients is taken into account.

7.15 It should be possible to sustain a capital programme for hospital develop-ment of about £9m annually (rather more than half the target level). This would allow both essential maintenance and upgrading in existing hospitals and also the provision of the better occupation and training facilities for in-patients which are central to rehabilitation.

7.16 The national projections given above tend inevitably—like others in this document—to mask the great diversity of local circumstances. Determining the order of priorities for any locality requires a full assessment of the existing services and needs. Collaboration and joint planning between health and local authorities are central to the success of the White Paper's aims and the maximum possible use should be made of the new joint financing arrangements.

Services for the Mentally Handicapped
Current Expenditure (£m November 1974 prices)

Figure 8

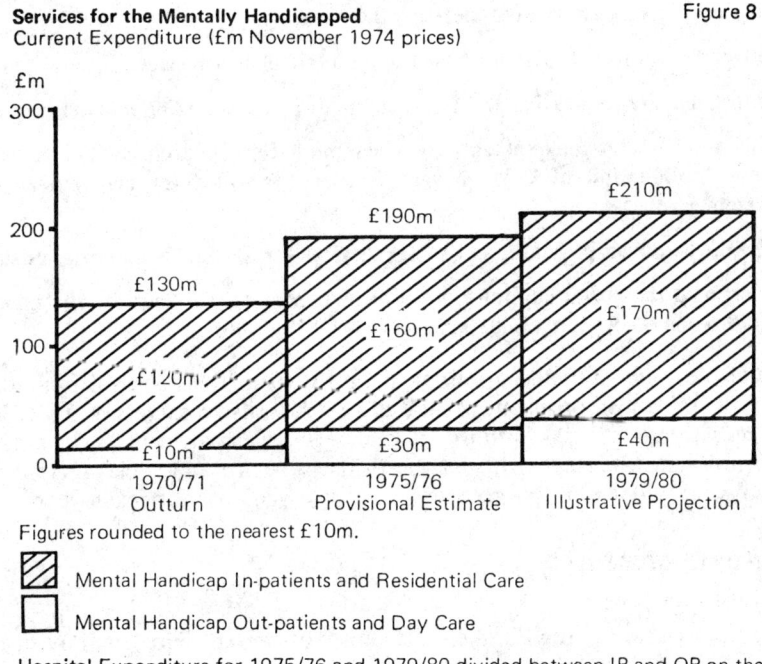

£m

1970/71 Outturn	1975/76 Provisional Estimate	1979/80 Illustrative Projection

Figures rounded to the nearest £10m.

Mental Handicap In-patients and Residential Care

Mental Handicap Out-patients and Day Care

Hospital Expenditure for 1975/76 and 1979/80 divided between IP and OP on the basis of OP increasing at £0.05m pa.

SERVICES FOR THE MENTALLY ILL

The Government's long-term strategy has been set out in the White Paper "Better Services for the Mentally Ill" (Cmnd 6233). The main services should be available locally in each district so that people can as far as possible receive treatment without losing touch with their usual life.

The priorities suggested to 1979/80 are:—

– the continued development of community care, with particular emphasis on low cost solutions. Increased capital programmes of £4m a year for day centres and £3m a year for residential accommodation are proposed. This would yield an additional 1,200 and 350 places a year respectively, though low cost approaches could increase the number.

– progress towards a District based psychiatric health service.

– improving staffing ratios and physical conditions in existing hospital services.

– the provision of adequate secure accommodation in each region. A special capital allocation of £2½m a year is being provided for regional security schemes.

– the development of health and social services for alcoholics and drug misusers.

It is proposed that total capital expenditure on hospital services for the mentally ill should reach the level of about £25m a year by 1979/80.

8.1 Each year an estimated 5 million people consult their general practitioner with a mental health problem. Mental ill-health is also a factor in many of the cases presenting to local authority social services departments. Most mental health problems are dealt with by the primary health and social services, but even so some 600,000 people receive specialist psychiatric care each year.

Long-term objectives

General strategy

8.2 Specialist services for the mentally ill are at present based mainly in large mental illness hospitals, often some distance from the communities they serve. The Government's long-term strategy for the further development of both health and personal social services is set out in the White Paper, *Better Services for the Mentally Ill* (Cmnd 6233) published in October, 1975. The main services needed by mentally ill people should be available locally in each district, so that people can as far as possible receive treatment while continuing to live at home. In-patient treatment in hospital, or residential care in a local authority home or hostel, should be provided only for those who cannot otherwise be helped effectively. The emphasis in such treatment and care should then be on helping the individual to cope with life in the community again to the fullest possible extent; even if a degree of more or less permanent support and care is needed the aim should be to give as much opportunity as possible for independence and self-fulfilment. The participation of family practitioner, social work and community nursing services is crucially important in these aims, as is the enlistment of voluntary help.

8.3 The elements of the strategy which can be separately costed are those involved in developing the range of specialist services. For these, the broad objectives set by the White Paper over the next 25 years are:—

- to increase local authority social services residential and day facilities, fieldwork, and domiciliary care, for the mentally ill. At present these fall far short of what is needed, so that many patients stay unnecessarily in hospital or are discharged to unsatisfactory conditions in the community.

- to provide locally based district hospital services, including a psychiatric department, as part of the district general hospital complex, for in-patient and day-patient treatment, and a community hospital unit for the elderly severely mentally infirm, together with regional and sub-regional units for certain special groups of patients, and units for the treatment of children and adolescents.

- to raise staffing ratios, particularly for medical, nursing and social work staff, and to develop the participation of and a close relationship with area social work teams and primary care staff in the care of the mentally ill. Also to improve standards through more and better training of both new and existing staff.

- pending the remodelling of the hospital services, to continue to raise standards in existing mental illness hospitals.

The last of these objectives is especially significant. The closure of mental illness hospitals is *not* in itself an objective of Government policy, and the White Paper stresses that hospitals should not encourage patients to leave unless there are satisfactory arrangements for their support. The possibility of closing a hospital depends both on the existence of the necessary range of health and local authority facilities, and on the length of time for which care must be provided for the hospital's remaining long-stay patients.

Long-stay patients

8.4 The network of district services is intended to take over from the mental hospitals the care and treatment of new patients. It is not intended – and the scale of facilities proposed would not enable it – to take over responsibility for the diminishing group of "old long-stay" patients. The development of modern and more active services is likely to reduce greatly the number of patients requiring long-term residential care. The White Paper discusses provision for this relatively small "new long-stay" group which might take the form of "hospital hostel" accommodation, for those who require 24 hour specialist nursing care and medical oversight, supplemented by long-stay local authority accommodation.

Elderly people with mental infirmity

8.5 There is a close interdependence, which is recognised in the Mental Illness White Paper, between services for the mentally ill and those for old people with mental infirmity, whose needs are discussed in Section V dealing with services for the elderly. This applies particularly to the elderly severely mentally infirm – those old people who need continuing hospital care (usually as a result of bementia) but do not require the treatment facilities of a mental illness hospital or unit. At present these patients are often cared for in mental hospitals, and paragraph 5.27 above explains how progress with plans for the mental illness services depends on progress in providing proper services for them in community hospital units, residential accommodation or other forms of care as appropriate.

Security

8.6 There is a serious shortage of facilities for patients needing treatment under conditions of greater security than is available in most psychiatric hospital units but less than the maximum security of the Special Hospitals. This has evoked severe criticism from the Courts and the public. Regional security units need to be established urgently as an integral part of the general psychiatric services for a region, and as centres for the development of a forensic psychiatric service; special funds have now been set aside for this purpose (see paragraph 8.19).

Alcoholism and drug misuse

8.7 Estimates of the prevalence of alcoholism suggest that in a health district of 250,000 population there may be some 2,000 adults with a serious drink problem, and that the number is growing, particularly among young people and women. There are specialised treatment units in most Regions (22 altogether) but these treat only a relatively small proportion of patients. Services at the local level are far less developed than psychiatric services generally. Related community services, where they exist, stem from voluntary effort and may be precariously financed. The prime objective is to move towards a more locally based approach with a multi-disciplinary team led by a consultant psychiatrist with a part-time special interest in alcoholism, using and supporting the skills of primary care teams, social workers and probation officers, and the resources of voluntary groups, and focussing on out-patient, day-patient or community facilities. In districts with many homeless alcoholics, hostels and other specialised services with access to detoxification facilities will be needed. It is also hoped to complete the network of specialised treatment units as a regional focus for experiment and training.

8.8 There are now few areas without some problem of drug misuse, but treatment services are still not available everywhere and in London they are overloaded. Help for non-narcotic drug misusers is patchy at best and voluntary community care facilities suffer from isolation and insecure finances. The objective is to involve health and local authorities in remodelling services, including the voluntary services, on a more local basis, responsive to local need and integrated with other services for young people.

Cost of implementation

8.9 The White Paper concluded that the cost of running the new services for the mentally ill should not, in the long run, be very different from that of continuing the existing pattern. The increase in professional staff would be offset to some degree by the reduction in the number of in-patients: the eventual reduction in total current costs on the health side would be balanced by an increase (already beginning) on the personal social services side. The capital cost of new health service provision over a 20/30 year period was estimated at £30m a year (including the necessary upgrading of mental hospitals in the interim and the cost of accommodation for the elderly severely mentally infirm). In real terms this is equivalent to the amount actually spent in 1972/73, which represented about 8 per cent of total hospital capital expenditure in that year; but by the following year both the amount, in real terms, and the share for mental illness had dropped. On the social services side the capital requirement over a 20/30 year period was estimated at £8m a year. This may be compared with about £3m actually spent in 1974/75. The latter sum was only 4 per cent of all personal social services capital expenditure and (though a higher percentage than any previous figure) was much less than the 10 per cent share advocated in the Department's guidance to local authorities for that year.

Priorities to 1979/80

8.10 We regard the development of services for the mentally ill as a major priority. The following paragraphs suggest how resources should be distributed between the different services required. The proposed rate of development would, if maintained, enable the aims of *Better Services for the Mentally Ill* to be achieved over most of the country within 25 years.

Community services

8.11 The most serious deficiencies in existing services for the mentally ill are in the local authority social services, where in 1974 there were fewer than 4,000 residential places, and only just over 5,000 day places, against an estimated national requirement of 12,000 and 30,000 places respectively. This does not necessarily reflect a lack of concern by authorities, a good many of whom could point to mental illness schemes for which they had requested loan sanction in the past few years but which the central government of the day had felt unable to approve. Even with the prospect of a sharp reduction overall in local authority capital schemes, it is essential that capital expenditure for mental illness should be increased, not only as a proportion of the total but in absolute terms, if there is to be any real progress either in meeting existing urgent needs or in developing the new pattern of services.

8.12 There is especially urgent need for more *day care*, which is at present (as the above figures show) the least adequately provided of all services for the mentally ill. Its availability may be a critical factor in determining the success with which a person recovering from mental illness is able to readjust to life in the community. It is suggested that there should be an accelerated capital programme of some £4m annually (double the present level) to provide about 1,200 additional day places a year. This would make it possible to achieve the White Paper guideline roughly over a 25-year period and implies growth at 15 per cent annually in current expenditure on day care.

8.13 The need to develop a range of suitable *residential accommodation* in the community for people who have been mentally ill is scarcely less pressing, and for this also an increased capital programme is suggested—at £3m annually, representing (on present assumptions about capital unit costs) some 350 places a year. The growth rate in current expenditure would be 7 per cent annually.

8.14 For both day care and residential services (but especially the latter) faster growth could be achieved by concentrating on forms of provision with a lower capital cost, and it is hoped that authorities will use all the means in their power to increase their services to the maximum for each pound of capital available. This can be done, for example, by:

– the use of adapted rather than purpose-built accommodation, where suitable premises are available.

- for day centres, sharing facilities with other groups with similar needs to the mentally ill or making premises serve more than one function, for example as a day centre during the day and as a community centre or youth centre during the evening.

- for residential accommodation, the use of boarding out and supervised lodging schemes. These do not involve capital cost, though placement needs care and social work support needs to be available if required. Schemes may be successfully operated by voluntary organisations.

- fuller use by local authorities of places in voluntary associations' hostels, some of which are at present under-occupied as a result of authorities seeking to reduce their financial commitment. A permanent understanding with a voluntary hostel can be more helpful to both sides than purely ad hoc arrangements.

- the use of group homes and other forms of housing suitable for those who need an environment providing some support rather than a substantial degree of care. Since the Housing Act 1974 the subsidies and grants available for other forms of housing provided by housing authorities or housing associations extend also to the provision of communal accommodation such as hostels. This could be a useful area of work especially for those voluntary bodies which are, or can work in association with, registered housing associations.

Close contact between the health service and the social services department, and between both and voluntary organisations, is of supreme importance in providing an effective service within the resources available. The arrangements for joint financing of community social services schemes are particularly relevant to the development of services for the mentally ill.

Progress towards a district based psychiatric health service

8.15 The proposed capital programme of £25m annually for mental illness hospital services would permit some progress in developing district based services. Within this field, the priorities are:—

- in districts where plans are well advanced, the development of a full district service with a psychiatric unit (including a day hospital), out-patient facilities, and units for the elderly severely mentally infirm. In many instances existing hospital premises may, if suitable, be adapted to provide the service, at least temporarily, at substantially lower capital cost. If necessary an acute psychiatric unit may be developed initially with fewer beds than the full number required, providing that it forms part of an agreed plan for the whole future district service: in the long run all the acute beds should be on a single site. The Department is currently reviewing building design requirements.

- in the majority of districts where a full service cannot be developed in the shorter term, selective development should be possible of services which do not require a large capital outlay but can reduce admission to hospitals or permit earlier discharges—in particular day hospitals, and units for the elderly severely mentally infirm (for both of which adapted premises are often suitable) and community psychiatric nursing services. Here again it is essential to work within an agreed overall plan covering both hospital and social services.

Continued improvement of existing psychiatric services

8.16 For some years to come, the majority of psychiatric patients will be cared for in the existing mental hospitals. Priorities here are:—

- the achievement of the minimum standards for staff ratios, food, accommodation and facilities which were defined by the Department in 1972. Most hospitals have now met most of the minima, but there are still some important gaps—for example, patients without personal clothing. Attainment of minimum standards, where they have not been reached, is the highest priority for additional current expenditure;

- improvement of physical standards in hospitals;

- the improvement of staffing levels, which is an essential element in all the health service developments considered here. Whereas the minimum staffing standards mentioned above (which are a first priority) are expressed as ratios of staff to in-patients, overall staffing targets (as set out in the White Paper) are related to the more relevant criterion of district population. The priority for new consultant posts are those districts with a ratio of less than one consultant psychiatrist to 60,000 population. The short-term target for nurses is 85 per 100,000 population (of whom 60 per cent excluding teaching and administrative staff should be qualified), though staffing levels will tend to vary from district to district. Increases of other professional staff, such as psychologists, are also important.

8.17 A regional strategy for the future of mental illness hospitals (on the lines set out in the Appendix to the White Paper) is needed so that decisions can be reached on the hospitals, or parts of hospitals, to be replaced first, and improvements concentrated in those which are to remain for longer.

8.18 To achieve these improvements it is proposed that current expenditure on in-patient and out-patient services should increase at an annual rate of about 1.3 per cent in the period to 1979/80. The falling number of in-patients gives some further margin for improvement. Although the future reduction cannot be predicted with certainty, a rough estimate is that by 1979/80 the number of occupied beds may have fallen to some 75,000 from the 1974 level of about 90,000. On this basis there would be an overall increase of 4–5 per cent annually in current expenditure per occupied bed, including expenditure on mental illness hospitals, psychiatric units, the new units for the elderly severely mentally infirm and regional security units.

Secure accommodation

8.19 Without the urgent provision of adequate secure accommodation in each region, the "open door" approach to care and treatment may be jeopardised by the small minority of patients needing greater restriction. A special capital allocation of £2.5m a year is being provided for regional security schemes. Special assistance will also be provided with their revenue consequences.

Services for alcoholics and drug misusers

8.20 Current trends in the demand for treatment, and the growth in alcoholism and alcohol-related problems, suggest that authorities should start now to develop the kind of services described in paragraphs 8.7 and 8.8. Much of this could be done at relatively small cost. Gaps and problems in the services for drug misusers also call for early attention.

Health capital

8.21 It is proposed that capital expenditure on hospital services for the mentally ill should reach the level of about £25m annually in the period to 1979/80. This represents increased investment in mental illness services (though still below the 1972/73 level) at a time when capital expenditure generally will be falling, and, as indicated in paragraph 8.15, it would permit significant progress in the establishment of district services as well as the improvement of existing hospitals. The broad distribution of the £25m might be as follows:—

	£m
Community hospital units for the elderly severely mentally infirm	7
Maintenance/upgrading of old hospitals	5
Hospital hostels	$\frac{1}{2}$
Regional Security Units	$2\frac{1}{2}$
General hospital provision	10
	—
	25

Services for the Mentally Ill
Current Expenditure (£m November 1974 prices)

Figure 9

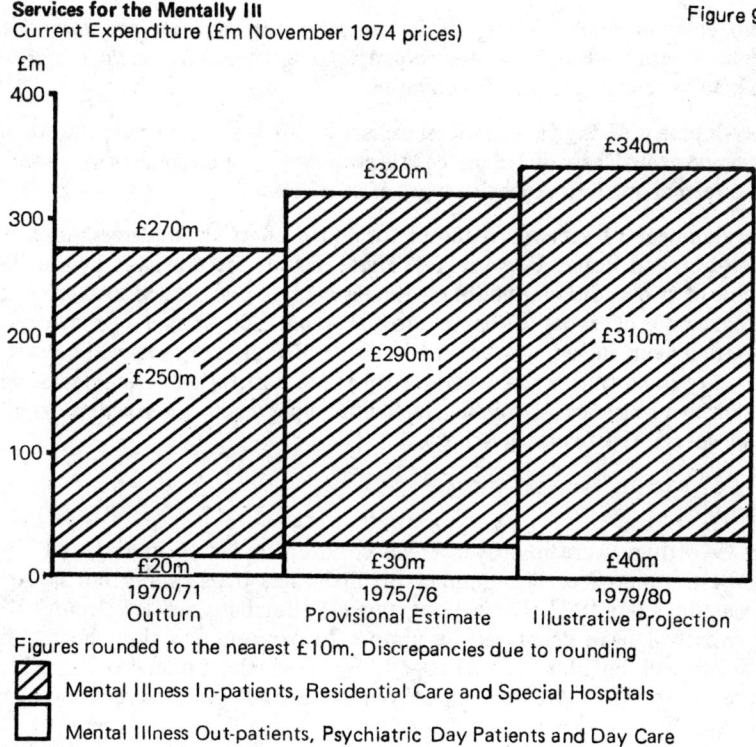

£m

Figures rounded to the nearest £10m. Discrepancies due to rounding

▨ Mental Illness In-patients, Residential Care and Special Hospitals

☐ Mental Illness Out-patients, Psychiatric Day Patients and Day Care

Hospital expenditure for 1975/76 and 1979/80 divided between IP and OP on basis of same growth rates for each as for total

IX

SERVICES FOR CHILDREN AND FAMILIES WITH CHILDREN

The health service needs of children include expert care at the time of birth and screening and surveillance during pre-school and school years. The main objective of the personal social services for children is to help families provide a satisfactory home for them, or where necessary to provide a substitute family or residential care. These services are under particular pressure from the growing number of children in trouble with the courts and the growing number who remain in care.

The priorities for the period to 1979/80 are:

– improvements in special care for babies in hospitals.

– expansion of health visiting services to allow for improvements in monitoring child health and welfare and support to mothers. An annual increase in expenditure of 6 per cent is proposed.

– development of day care services, especially for pre-school children. An annual revenue growth rate of $2 \cdot 5$ per cent is proposed, with an emphasis on developing less formal and less expensive types of provision.

– development of services required for more effective implementation of the Children and Young Persons Act. These include the provision by the Department of two additional youth treatment centres and a local authority capital programme of about £10m to provide about 500 special community home places a year, including secure places for which direct grants will be available. Equally important is the development of non-institutional methods of helping children at risk or in trouble, including supervision, intermediate treatment and specialised fostering schemes.

General

9.1 In 1973 there were just over $11\frac{1}{2}$m children under 16 in England, $3\frac{1}{2}$m of whom were under five. The number of births has been falling but is expected to rise again from 1977. Projections suggest that between 1973 and 1979 the under-fives will have decreased by almost 20 per cent but that the school age population will be almost unchanged. By 1985 the under-fives would have recovered to the 1973 level and the school-age group would have fallen by about 17 per cent.

9.2 The indicators of need tell a different and more disturbing story. Although infant mortality has been reduced, the improvement is far less rapid than in other developed countries. While it is not possible to infer any trends from statistics about the abuse and neglect of children by adults there is no mistaking the increase in public concern about it. The great majority of children in England are healthier than ever before. But for the same reasons children with mental and/or physical handicapping conditions are surviving well into the school years and beyond. Handicapped children are one of today's chief problems in child health.

9.3 The number of children under 17 found guilty of indictable offences, or who have admitted such offences without court proceedings being taken, has grown from 118,883 in 1970 to 184,491 in 1974. This is an average annual increase of 11·6 per cent. The number of children coming into care each year has remained fairly static at around 50,000 a year since 1964 but the number staying in care has steadily risen; as a result the total number in care has recently been rising at about 2·5 per cent a year.

9.4 Both health and personal social services for children aim to assist the full development of the child's physical, intellectual, emotional and social potentialities. Particular importance is attached to the perinatal period and the pre-school years which are of crucial importance for the child's later development.

Health services for children

9.5 In broad terms the health service needs of children are expert care at birth and during the first weeks of life; primary care and support, and screening programmes, during the pre-school and school years, to identify, as early as possible, deviant development of any kind; comprehensive assessment and follow-up of children thought or found to be handicapped in any way; and family doctor and hospital specialist care for the sick child with supporting care in the community on return home. The report of the committee under the chairmanship of Professor Court, covering the whole subject of health services for children, is expected in 1976. The cost of services provided specially or mainly for children—child health clinics, health visiting, the school health service—is estimated at just over £110m annually, of which about £50m is spent on school health services. Home nursing, used mainly by the elderly, is also a significant service for pre-school children. Welfare foods cost about £8m annually.

Hospital services

9.6 Policies on hospital services for children were set out in the report of the Expert Group on Special Care for Babies (1971) and in HM(71)22. There is an urgent need to improve the level of special care for low birthweight and sick newborn babies, so as to reduce still further the incidence of neonatal mortality and of chronic handicap. The Departmental target of 6 cots per 1,000 live births has been attained nationally but not in all Regions, and some further capital investment will be needed. It is estimated that an extra £1·0m current expenditure (mainly for extra medical and nursing staff) and £0·8m for equipment are needed nationally to bring the service up to an acceptable level. It is likely, however, that the improvement of staffing levels could only be achieved over a period of several years. There is also a priority need to develop comprehensive assessment and follow-up services to help handicapped children reach their full potential; at present only about 50 per cent of districts provide the service. An important part of the service is guidance and support for parents, including genetic counselling. The cost of expansion is hard to assess because much of the service would be provided by existing staff.

9.7 In 1974 over 800,000 children under 15 were treated as in-patients in hospitals in England, and there were about 4 million out-patient attendances. The DHSS has urged in HM(71)22 that children should wherever possible be treated as out-patients or day patients, and that when admitted to hospital they should as far as possible be accommodated in children's departments under the general oversight of a paediatrician. It has also emphasised the need to avoid keeping children in hospital for long periods. At present there is a considerable shortage of nurses with children's nursing qualifications.

Community health services

9.8 These services provide health support for families with young children, but less than half (about 46 per cent) of children under age five attend a child health clinic each year (though in addition an unknown number attend general practitioners' clinics). The National Children's Bureau publication "From Birth to Seven" suggested that families in social classes IV and V had the lowest rates of attendance. Health visitors can help to encourage greater use of clinic services and more health visitor time is also needed for routine home visits to all children—particularly those in the lower socio-economic groups—to provide support for the parents, to perform some screening tests in the home, and to observe the children's behaviour and development in their home environment. This is estimated to require an increase in the number of health visitors providing services for the under-fives from their present total of about 4,000 to over 7,000 (whole-time equivalent). Health visiting is a service which, imaginatively managed, can be very effectively deployed to help those most in need. Health visitors also have a crucial role in the prevention of non-accidental injury (see below). For both these reasons their expansion is a high priority.

9.9 The expansion of home nursing services (used mainly by the elderly) is also needed to enable children to be treated as far as possible in their own homes and reduce the numbers left in hospitals for long periods.

The school health service

9.10 The main objectives of child health services in relation to education are to provide continuing health surveillance of all children throughout the school years; to promote awareness among teachers and parents of the effect that medical, surgical and neurodevelopmental disorders of childhood may have on a child's ability to learn; and to contribute to health education. Central government policy for many years has been to discourage routine periodic examinations of children in particular age groups, and to encourage closer and more continuous links between health service staff and teachers. This should lead to better and more economical use of staff. An immediate priority should be to maintain and consolidate services as far as resources permit pending the report of the Child Health Service Committee. Deterioration of services and of staff morale while "waiting for Court" would be very expensive to correct.

Personal social services for children

9.11 It is a key objective of the personal social services to support the family. Where children are concerned the main objective is to help families provide a satisfactory home for the child, and to enable children to stay with their families except where it is against the children's interests. Many of the services provided specifically for children are required when the child's home no longer provides a satisfactory environment, either temporarily or permanently, or when the child has no family of his own, and it is necessary to provide a substitute family or, in some cases, residential care. The main interest at present is, however, in developing forms of help which minimise the need to take the child away from the family.

9.12 The local authority social services for children include residential care, fostering, adoption services, support for parents and children in the home, day nurseries and other forms of day care for pre-school children, and play groups.

The pivot of all these services is the social worker. This is particularly true where the help provided takes the form (as increasingly it should) of support in the home. But social work is also a vital element in the other services mentioned—in assessing needs for residential and other forms of care; in maintaining contact with families; in supervising standards of fostering.

9.13 Because the social work element cannot be separately costed, expenditure figures for the services do not give a complete picture. Expenditure which can be identified separately is estimated as about £110m annually on residential care, £20m on day nurseries and pre-school play groups, and £14m on boarding out.

9.14 The Children and Young Persons Act, 1969, transferred to the social services a number of important and expensive services which were previously seen as part of the law and order services. It set out to integrate services for young people who commit offences more closely with those provided for children generally, including residential services, services for children under court orders and the new concept of intermediate treatment. The 1969 Act has substantially increased the work load of the personal social services and the demands on their resources. This has been obvious in the case of residential care, but it is important to remember that successful use of the other services for children can reduce demand for residential places later on (see paragraph 9.18).

Support in the home

9.15 Both the NHS and the personal social services provide support for parents and children in the home. Health visitors probably visit more families with children than any other profession. The width of their responsibilities (as well as staff shortages) limits the depth of their involvement, but they are well placed to see danger signs and alert other services where appropriate. In field social work, preventive work aimed at reducing the number of children coming into care needs to be further developed. This is a vital area for inter-professional co-operation and planning, which are also critically important in tackling the problem of non-accidental injury to children. These cases highlight a general need for expansion of social work, health visiting and other relevant services; an immediate short-term priority is to improve communications between different individuals and authorities concerned with the child. All local authorities in England have now established Area Review Committees as policy-making bodies for case management and it is hoped that registers of children at risk, which have been started by many authorities, will soon be set up in all areas.

Day care

9.16 Day care for pre-school children has an essential role in alleviating the effects of social deprivation in the child's formative years. Local authority facilities are concentrated on those who have priority need, and they have long waiting lists. Private arrangements, voluntary agencies and employers provide a significant and growing proportion of day care services, for example playgroups and childminders. Up to now new local authority building has been at the rate of about 1,000-2,000 additional places a year but the present financial constraints point to slower expansion and there are staffing problems. In the private sector many children are being placed with unregistered minders about whose standards of care little is known. Experiment with informal and less expensive types of local authority day care, which might enable the most urgent needs to be met more quickly and may be preferable on child care grounds, is a high priority— as is co-ordination of all services for pre-school children at local level, including health support. Substantial support is needed for the expanding playgroup movement.

Fostering

9.17 The development of alternatives to institutional treatment for children and young people in trouble with the courts is a main objective of the 1969 Act. Fostering or boarding out can provide for many children an alternative to residential care which is preferable on grounds both of cost and of the nature of the care provided. In March 1974 there were 29,400 children boarded out by local authorities in England. It has been estimated that a further 5,000 or so children living in residential homes at an average cost of around £50 a week to local authorities could be boarded out, if suitable foster parents could be found, at less cost. More social work time would, however, be taken up in arranging placements. Many authorities are trying to improve recruitment and fostering standards, and improvements are also needed in the notification and supervision of private fostering arrangements.

Supervision and intermediate treatment

9.18 The 1969 Act provides for court supervision orders under which it is the duty of the supervisor "to advise, assist and befriend" a child or young person for up to three years. Responsibility for supervision is being gradually transferred from the probation service to local authorities. In 1974 the latter became responsible for supervising children under 13. The estimated additional case-load is about 2,000 children. A further transfer in 1975 was postponed, however. Reports suggest an urgent need to improve the quality of supervision. The rough estimate that 60,000 children are subject to supervision orders indicates the substantial demand supervision orders make on social workers' time. A professional estimate is that each case might require two hours a week of a social worker's time in the first year, reducing to one hour in the second and half an hour in the third year. This level of attention would require about 2,000 social workers full time, or one-sixth of all field social workers—a clear illustration of the gap between expectations and resources. The Act also enables courts to add to a supervision order provisions requiring a child to take part in approved activities (intermediate treatment) under the direction of the supervisor or in short residential courses. Latest reports indicate growing interest in intermediate treatment but much uncertainty about how to operate it. The Social Work Service are giving high priority to its development and guidance on policy and financial aspects is in preparation.

Residential care

9.19 Meanwhile there is substantial unmet need for residential care. This may to some extent be due to unsatisfactory use of the places which are available. But some homes are badly run-down, others are in the wrong place—too far away from the communities they serve—and there are serious shortages of specialised accommodation, particularly secure accommodation, both for remands and for treatment. Growing numbers of young people, including 14 year old girls, are having to be remanded to prison service establishments because secure community home places are not available (there were 3,889 such remands in 1974). Even after the reduction in key sector building plans following the 1975 budget, local authorities received provisional approval to spend £18m on community homes (including 1,838 new places of which 155 are secure).

9.20 Three youth treatment centres are being developed, as a direct responsibility of the Department, for the small minority of highly disturbed children who cannot reasonably be accommodated in community homes. One centre is in operation, a second is being built and it is hoped that all three will be completed by 1978, providing a total of 188 places. A characteristic of the centres is the very high ratio of staff to children: it is estimated that the three centres will require a total of 250 professional staff, including residential social workers, nurses and teachers. This represents a significant demand on national resources, but there are some indications even at this stage that the centres can play an effective part in preventing the drift of disturbed adolescents into a lifetime in prisons or mental hospitals.

Implementation of the Children Act 1975

9.21 Additional responsibilities, notably in the field of adoption, will fall upon local authorities by the implementation of the Children Act 1975 but it has been accepted that the rate at which its provisions will be implemented must take account of local authority resources. A number of provisions can be implemented in 1976/77 within existing resources. In the summer of 1976 Ministers will be reviewing, in consultation with local authorities, the pace of implementation for the bulk of the Act. The major demand for additional money and manpower will arise from the development of comprehensive local authority adoption services and it is clear that the statutory duty to provide these cannot be introduced before 1978/79 at the earliest. The provision for separate representation of children in care and related proceedings would represent a less substantial call on resources and it is hoped that some of these provisions can be implemented at an early date.

Suggested developments to 1979/80

9.22 There are obvious reasons why services for children must in principle command a high priority. However, during the next few years it will not be possible for expenditure to increase as rapidly as in the past. In proposing the level of resources to be allocated to children's services the attempt has been made to identify the key points where needs are most pressing. Although there will be some benefit to the services from the fall in the child population, this is qualified by the uneven pattern of the projected changes.

9.23 Generally it must be emphasised that the various expenditure projections given in this document are only a partial guide to relative priorities in services for children. There are key developments in the hospital services which cannot be separately costed at present, and in the personal social services field the emphasis on non-institutional solutions represents an additional call on social work services which does not appear in the residential and day care projections.

9.24 It is proposed that the first priority should be the improvement, in places where facilities are currently inadequate, of *special care for newborn babies*, where there is the potential both to save lives and to improve greatly the quality of life by preventing lifelong handicap. This service forms part of the acute hospital services and is not separately costed, but the urgent improvements mentioned above (paragraph 9.5) could be achieved at a relatively small cost.

9.25 Expansion of the *health visiting service*, with its crucial role in protecting the health of the most vulnerable children and bringing to notice cases of neglect and ill-treatment, is also a key priority. Faster growth than in the recent past is justified and we propose a 6 per cent annual increase in expenditure on the service. Among the other community health services, children would also benefit from the 6 per cent growth rate in home nursing proposed in the context of services for the elderly (paragraph 5.15). Current expenditure on clinics is projected to remain constant (provision of clinic services will increase with the relatively rapid growth in health centres) as is that on the school health service (where the projected 17 per cent fall by 1985 in the 5-15 age group points to restraint).

9.26 It is suggested that another priority should be the expansion of *day care services*, especially for children in the pre-school age group. The current expenditure annual growth rate of 2·5 per cent and the capital expenditure of £1m projected here are modest and would allow the provision of only about 400 day nursery places annually—not enough to meet priority needs for many years to come. The scope for development depends in large part on the more informal kinds of provision mentioned above and on the enlistment and maximum use of voluntary help.

9.27 The continued development of the pattern of services required for more effective implementation of the Children and Young Persons Act 1969 is another priority task. There is an urgent need for *secure accommodation* both for remands, so that young people do not have to be remanded to prison, and for long-term control and treatment. The Department will be maintaining its programme for providing two more youth treatment centres. A programme of 100 per cent grants to local authorities, which was recently announced, should enable them to build roughly an additional 100 places a year at an annual cost of about £2m. This might form part of a capital programme of some £10m to provide about 500 mainly special (including secure) community home places annually and implies an average growth rate of 2·5 per cent in current expenditure on community homes to 1979/80.

9.28 A residential programme on this scale will leave little room for expansion of community homes outside the special and secure categories, and it will be important to develop the alternative approaches mentioned in this section to the extent that the availability of social work support permits. A special priority is the development of intermediate treatment and other forms of non-residential treatment for children in trouble or at risk.

Conclusion

9.29 1976 seems likely to be a critical year for the children's services. Policy in relation to the 1969 Act and to day care is under review as this document is written. In both cases there is strong public demand to reproduce old patterns of institutional provision, and too little understanding of the difficulties of operating children's homes and day nurseries in changed conditions, or the shortcomings in the care they can provide. Large numbers of staff are required to run children's homes and day nurseries; residential care particularly is unattractive as a career to young people nowadays; and our expectations about standards make these institutions disproportionately expensive. Their cost alone

Services Mainly for Children
Current Expenditure (£m November 1974 prices)   Figure 10

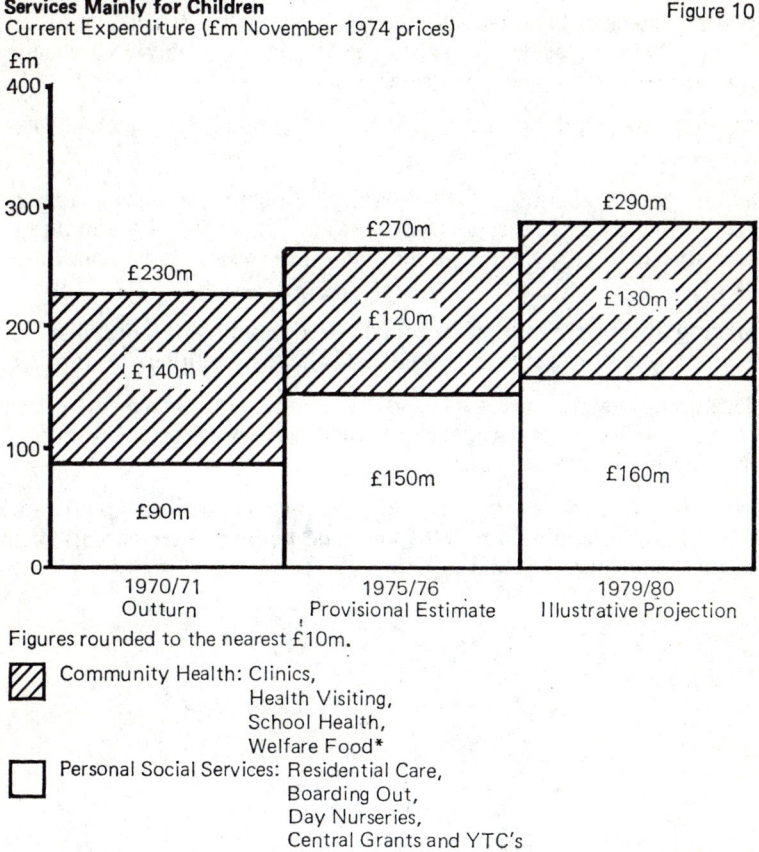

£m

Figures rounded to the nearest £10m.

Community Health: Clinics,
                 Health Visiting,
                 School Health,
                 Welfare Food*

Personal Social Services: Residential Care,
                         Boarding Out,
                         Day Nurseries,
                         Central Grants and YTC's

* £40m fall in Welfare Food between 1970/71 and 1975/76

rules out any possibility that demand could be met. Despite the growing demand in both fields new building over the past five years has probably done little more than replace buildings that have ceased to be usable. These are fields in which imaginative new policies to meet real needs could be put into operation without additional public expenditure. Similar dilemmas can be seen in the health field, where the report of the Committee on the Child Health Services is expected this year.

9.30 The critical constraint in developing the new policies that are needed is the shortage of trained staff. But the child is in the community now. So are his parents. If they cannot get professional help they have to manage on their own with what help and advice they can get from friends, relations and neighbours. Leaving aside the special problems of cruelty and neglect, the situation seems to demand such strategies as:

– using ancillary and voluntary workers to economise on scarce professional resources;

– making maximum use of community resources such as foster parents, child minders and the often forgotten aunts and grandmothers (who probably meet a great part of the nation's needs for day care and foster care);

– making maximum use of voluntary and community organisations, for example the playgroup movement and the local mothers' groups;

– developing new resources such as day centres and intermediate treatment centres which can make full use of staff who are not attracted to professional training in the caring professions;

– exploring the use of the media to supplement professional work, for example by providing advice to mothers, finding foster parents or helping to raise standards of child minding.

X

PERSONAL SOCIAL SERVICES

This section comments briefly on important general aspects of the personal social services and summarises the implications for these services of the proposals in earlier sections.

The role of social services departments

10.1 As the preceding sections have stressed, personal social services have an essential and increasing part to play in meeting the needs of particular client groups. But they also have wider responsibilities. The philosophy of the Seebohm Report, and of the Local Authority Social Services Act 1970 which established the new local authority departments, was that services should be developed to identify and respond to the differing needs of families and individuals in the community, irrespective of how they arose. The client groups specifically considered in this document by no means account for all the community's needs for personal social services. Families in need of help often present a mixture of problems which sometimes find expression in marital violence, alcoholism, juvenile delinquency, or in other ways. The personal social services have to decide how to respond to a large and varied range of problems which are themselves interwoven with forces affecting society more widely. The establishment of social services departments has—as it was meant to— brought these problems much more fully into the light. The new departments have greater scope for preventive work to reduce the incidence of family breakdown, homelessness, delinquency and child neglect and to reduce also the need for reception into residential or hospital care. Legislation has added to the opportunities and pressures, notably the Children and Young Persons Act and the Chronically Sick and Disabled Persons Act (mentioned in previous sections) and the National Health Service Reorganisation Act, which made them responsible for social work support for the health service.

10.2 To cope with these wider responsibilities and with the client group needs described in earlier sections, personal social services have in recent years expanded very rapidly (though from a relatively small base). Given the Government's conclusion in the Public Expenditure White Paper (Cmnd 6393) that no increase in the total of local authority current expenditure can be afforded over the next few years, it is clear that it will not be possible for expansion of the services to continue at anything like the recent rate. But as far as is possible within the financial constraints, the continuing pressures on these services are reflected in the proposals in this document.

Joint planning

10.3 The emphasis in previous sections has necessarily been on establishing planning priorities for the working partnership between social services departments and the NHS. But personal social services have equally important links with other local authority services (notably education and housing), as well as close working relationships with agencies outside local government (such as the Department's own local social security offices and the probation and employment services). Planning of health and personal social services has to be properly related to local authority corporate planning, and will be assisted by a national joint approach to social policy. The Government have made

71

clear their commitment to this approach and readiness to co-operate in any way they can in removing administrative barriers to effective action, or in re-assessing priorities for centrally provided services. Some of the basic problems which lie at the root of demands for personal social services are also being tackled by the Government in a variety of other ways—in particular, by regularly uprating social security benefits, by introducing new benefits, and by using all practicable means to improve the take-up of benefits, as well as by encouraging the provision of local authority housing at a cost which, with rebates, all can meet.

Community support

10.4 A further important general aspect of the work of social services departments is the link with community activity. Voluntary organisations have a particularly important role in engaging the help of a wider range of community resources. Liaison with them, and work with volunteers, require social service staff time, but support for voluntary effort and encouragement of self-help schemes may represent better value for money than directly provided services and may also provide the means of continuing preventive work. By their diversity and the ingenuity they bring to the task, voluntary organisations can be an important adjunct to the authority's own direct services in getting help to people in need.

Manpower and training

10.5 We propose that a key element in the general strategy for personal social services should be to increase the level of training and to improve the use made of skilled manpower. There is a particular scarcity of trained staff; among field social workers, in 1974, out of about 11,800 whole time and 1,700 part-time staff, the numbers with a professional qualification in social work were only about 4,500 and 600 respectively. The proportion is much lower in day care and residential care; in residential care in particular, only about 4 per cent of all staff have a relevant professional qualification, most of these being concentrated in homes for children and young people. At the same time, it is known that much of the time of professionally qualified workers is occupied in tasks which do not require their skills. Present pressures make it all the more important to use these skills where they are really needed, and to delegate more routine functions to less qualified workers.

10.6 The importance of developing training for the personal social services has been recognised by Government, the local authority associations, the Central Council for Education and Training in Social Work, and the Personal Social Services Council. A National Working Party on Manpower and Training for Social Services, including representatives of these and other interested bodies, has been considering the desirable rate and direction of development of training, and has recently reported to Ministers. Its report, which will be made generally available in the near future, stresses the need for economical and appropriate use of scarce resources of manpower, and recommends further development of:—

- basic qualifying training for the personal social services, especially for residential and day care;
- specialised post-qualifying training; and
- training for the effective management of the personal social services.

72

The Working Party also recommends that central and local government should at the earliest opportunity jointly review the arrangements for the financing of training. The White Paper on Public Expenditure to 1979/80 indicates that there should be room for some expenditure on the training recommendations of the Working Party, and in the proposals summarised below an allowance of £6m by 1979/80 has accordingly been made for the first phase of implementing these recommendations.

Summary of proposals for personal social services

10.7 The proposals for personal social services are summarised in Annex 2, Table 2. They are based on the estimate for these services in the Public Expenditure White Paper with the addition of the joint financing money for community social services referred to in paragraph 1.15. The actual level of expenditure will depend on the decisions of individual local authorities and, in the case of joint finance, on agreement with the corresponding health authority.

10.8 Table 2 of Annex 2 shows an overall rate of growth of *current* expenditure (excluding loan charges) of 2·9 per cent a year up to 1979/80, assuming a contribution of £12m from joint financing by health authorities. This is made up of an annual increase in expenditure on residential care of about 2·6 per cent, on day care (where total expenditure is much less) of about 5 per cent, and on boarding out, home helps, meals services and field social work of 2 per cent. To this has to be added the £6m allowance for social work training mentioned in paragraph 10.6 and an additional £5m on aids, adaptations and other services for the disabled.

10.9 The proposed annual level of *capital* expenditure for 1979/80 is £59m. This assumes the continuation of a fairly steady rate of capital investment from 1977/78 after a sharp fall from the estimated 1975/76 level of £100m. The £59m includes an estimated contribution of £15m by health authorities under the proposed joint financing arrangements.

10.10 The percentage distribution, between different services, of the capital expenditure suggested in this document for 1979/80 (as summarised in Annex 2, Table 2), compared with the estimated figures for 1975/76, would be as follows:—

Percentage of total PSS capital expenditure (excluding land, vehicles, etc.)

	1975/76 (estimated) per cent	1979/80 (suggested) per cent
Elderly and physically handicapped:		
Residential	41	30
Day care	10	2
Mental handicap:		
Residential	10	20
Day care	9	12

	1975/76 (estimated) per cent	1979/80 (suggested) per cent
Mental illness:		
Residential	2	6
Day care	2	8
Children:		
Residential	21	20
Day nurseries	3	2

10.11 The order of priorities which this document proposes in national terms is not, however, meant to be mirrored in each locality, for the reasons mentioned in the Introduction. There are some general principles reflected in these proposals to which the Government attach considerable importance, and for which they hope there will be general acceptance—for example the improvement of levels of community care for the mentally ill and mentally handicapped. However, the detailed figures given here represent only one possible pattern of development based on this general scale of priorities. Local authorities, in consultation with health authorities, will want to consider this in the light of local needs, the level of existing services, their statutory duties and their responsibilities to the local electorate.

10.12 One of the main issues for local and national consideration is whether, and if so, how, it is possible to make room for a higher rate of expansion of domiciliary and fieldwork services which is as desirable on broad grounds of policy as for economic reasons. Should it for example be sought by further reduction of the residential capital programme, by reduction in unit costs where these are relatively high, by reduction of administrative overheads, or in other ways?

10.13 Local authorities and their staff will need to continue and where possible intensify the efforts they have been making to secure more effective use of resources. But, however successful their efforts, adjustment to more modest levels of growth will undoubtedly be difficult for social services departments, and the Government accept that it will not be possible in the foreseeable future to meet in full all the needs which have progressively come to light. Authorities and their staffs will continue to have hard judgements to make between needs which it is essential for the services to meet, and those which individuals and families must themselves be left to cope with. The development of a manageable order of priorities also requires recognition on the part of the community generally that there are limits to what the social services can do to alleviate social need.

XI

1980-1985

11.1 In this section we set out briefly the general considerations as we see them which might affect the use of resources by the various programmes and services in the years after 1980. The Government hope that by 1980 the economy will have improved, and that a higher resource allocation will be available for the social programmes than is possible at present. On the other hand the economic situation might require a growth rate for health and personal social services similar to, or lower than, that proposed up to 1979/80.

11.2 The policies and objectives outlined in previous sections will need to continue in the period up to 1985 and beyond. The general aim will be to make as much progress as possible towards these objectives within the limits of overall resources. There are, however, too many uncertainties to allow more specific national objectives to be set, and we do not give any illustrative growth projections beyond 1980.

11.3 In addition to the difficulty of predicting the level of resources that will be available, there are uncertainties about demographic trends (in particular the number of births and hence of children), and about developments in patterns of treatment and care. The balance of priorities will also depend on progress made in the planning and development of services and the redeployment of resources in the period up to 1980. Subject to these uncertainties, we propose that the broad priorities outlined in earlier sections should be continued, but the balance may need to be adjusted to take account of the factors discussed below.

Demography

11.4 The number of elderly people will continue to increase, though as a whole the increase will be less than in the next few years because the number of people in the 65–74 age group will fall. However, the number of people aged 75 and over will continue to increase (at around 1·8 per cent a year), and since it is they who have the largest need for services, those programmes which provide care and treatment for the elderly will continue to face increasing pressures, and are likely to require a significant proportion of any available growth. The number of women of child bearing age is also increasing, and if, as suggested in the "central projection" of the Office of Population Censuses and Surveys, the birth rate increases as well, the number of births and children under five will rise rapidly. In this case services for younger children and families, and perhaps also the maternity services, will need to expand if standards are to be maintained. If on the other hand the birth rate follows the OPCS "continuing low" projection, then the number of births and children under five may remain below the 1973 level, and the number of children may continue to fall. In this case, there may be scope for further reduction in the maternity services, and for some economies in the health services used by children; however, the number of children in care, and families needing support, may continue to rise even if the birth rate remains low.

Primary care services

11.5 We expect that expenditure on the family practitioner services will continue to increase fairly rapidly, although the growth should be a little slower than in the years to 1980 because by then it is expected that expenditure on family planning will have stabilised. We propose that the health centre programme should continue.

General and acute hospital services

11.6 It is likely that the need to cater for new methods of treatment will be no less in the next decade than it is in the present one; and the use of these services by people over 75 will continue to grow. The scope for rationalising patterns of provision and increasing efficiency will depend in part on the progress that has been made in the intervening years. If measures of rationalisation and increased efficiency have been carried through effectively by the end of the decade, the scope for further redeployment and improvement in resource use will be less. There may, therefore, be a case for giving these services a larger share of any available growth after 1980 than we suggest for them in the intervening years.

Services for particular client groups

11.7 The priorities suggested to 1980 would allow some development of services for the mentally ill and the mentally handicapped. In order to promote a shift in the patterns of care consistent with the White Paper targets there would be a continuing need for capital and current expenditure on the appropriate personal social services; higher capital expenditure on remodelling hospital services would also be necessary. This would obviously depend on the growth in resources. As already mentioned the increasing number of elderly will continue to put heavy demands on the personal social services, and if the birthrate increases the services for children will also need expansion.

Other factors

11.8 If more resources were available, there would be a strong case for increasing the general hospital capital programme to allow more progress on building new hospitals and other developments. There are also a number of specific policies which we should like to carry out in the early 1980s if sufficient resources were available. Notable among these is implementation of the Briggs report on nurse training which, as stated in section II, is estimated to cost £27m a year once it has got under way.

11.9 If the economic situation improved and there were—say—a rate of annual growth in real terms resources after 1980 about double the rate that there will be for the rest of this decade, there would be scope for progress in most of the priority areas, by contrast with the emphasis on maintaining standards over the next four years. If, however, no greater growth could be made available to the services after 1980—or the rate of growth were even below the rate up to 1980—the range of choice would appear very limited. There would seem on that hypothesis to be little option but to make do with existing old buildings and to distribute any small amount of additional resources that might become available in the light of the most urgent needs as they appeared at the time, including the needs of the growing numbers of people over 75.

Home Population England
(1974 based projections)
1973 = 100

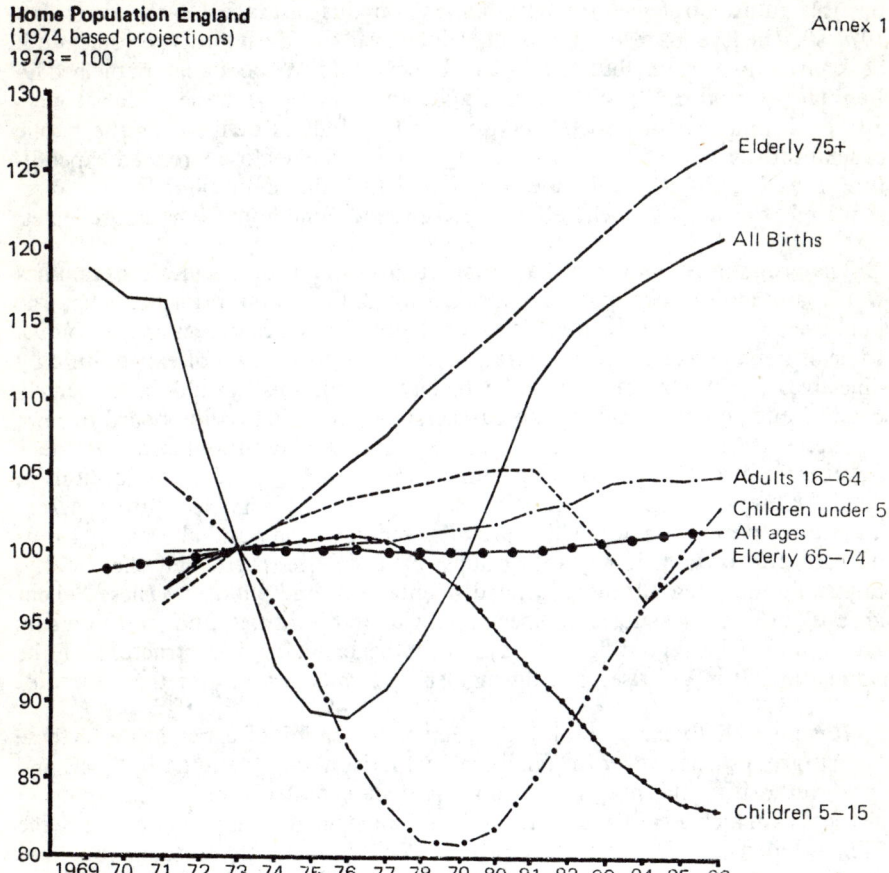

130

125 — Elderly 75+

120 — All Births

115

110

105 — Adults 16–64
Children under 5
100 — All ages
Elderly 65–74

95

90

85 — Children 5–15

80
1969 70 71 72 73 74 75 76 77 78 79 80 81 82 83 84 85 86

THE PROGRAMME BUDGET: NOTE ON METHOD AND SUMMARY TABLES

1. The programme budget is not a complex technical tool but a crude method of costing policies based on past expenditure. Its central purpose is to enable the Department to cost policies for service development across the board, so that priorities can be considered within realistic financial constraints. The programme budget is neither a forecast nor a plan: it is a way of exploring possible future strategies for development, in this instance for the period to 1979/80. The level of resources which will be available during this period cannot be known for certain, but the Public Expenditure White Paper published in February (Cmnd 6393) offers a firm guideline. The programme budget covers all health and personal social services for England, as defined for the public expenditure survey, at a national aggregate level. Some closely related expenditure is excluded because it does not fall within this definition, for instance, sheltered housing, and sheltered employment and blind home workers' schemes.

2. The programme budget also attempts to group expenditure into programmes which are more meaningful in considering options and priorities than the public expenditure survey breakdown or the traditional estimates and accounts. In health and personal social services a complete breakdown of expenditure by objectives (eg treatment of specific medical conditions) would be extremely detailed and complex, and far too cumbersome for an across-the-board review; the necessary data is not in any case available. The programme budget does not therefore contain the kind of information needed for evaluating options in detail. However, there are certain major groups of services cutting across administrative boundaries, which provide complementary and alternative forms of care for certain important groups of users, in particular the elderly, physically and mentally handicapped, mentally ill and children. These "client groups" are also the subject of special policies and priorities, and their numbers are changing in very different ways with the changing age structure of the population. It is also useful to distinguish maternity services for these reasons.

3. It is possible to carry out a fairly detailed allocation of expenditure to these "client groups". However, to facilitate comparison with planning by NHS and local authorities, the programmes in this document are simply a grouping of services by major user. Thus for instance all home nursing and geriatric medicine are included in the "elderly" programme, and health visiting (but not paediatrics, which cannot be costed separately) under "children"; primary care and hospital services used by the whole population (including the elderly and children) are shown as two separate "whole population" programmes, and maternity services are identified separately within the hospital services programme. There is so much overlap between services for the elderly and physically handicapped that these have been grouped together. The resulting grouping is shown in Table 1 at the end of this Annex; an alternative grouping, following administrative boundaries, is at Table 2.

4. As a starting point for costing future policy, past trends in expenditure are examined. For this document, the four years 1970/71 to 1973/74 are considered. For the family practitioner, centrally financed, ex-local health and personal

social services, expenditure figures are available from the appropriation and local authority accounts. These outturn figures are converted to 1975 survey (ie November 1974) prices, and certain other adjustments are made (eg income with the netted off and local authority debt charges removed) in accordance with the public expenditure survey costing conventions. For personal social services administrative costs are allocated to services.

5. For hospital services, a method of breaking down current expenditure has been developed on the basis of the accounts and hospital costing returns* before reorganisation. (With some modification the same method can be used with the new form of accounts and costing returns). Briefly, the expenditure in the costing returns is adjusted by adding in type 19(i) hospitals, dental hospitals and clinics, and this total is split into in-patients, out-patients and day patients. Day patient expenditure is subdivided into psychiatric and non-psychiatric day patients. For in-patients and out-patients, unit costs are derived from the costing returns as follows:—

Geriatric and younger disabled IP bed weeks and OP attendances: Regional Hospital Board Types 6 and 19(ii) (weighted average).
Mental illness IP bed weeks and OP attendances: RHB Type 12.
Mental handicap IP bed weeks and OP attendances: RHB Type 13.
Maternity IP cases and OP attendances: RHB Type 11.

These unit costs are then applied to all bed weeks, cases or attendances in the SH3 returns to give total expenditure for each item. The remaining expenditure in the RHB hospitals is then attributed to all other IP cases and OP attendances (broadly described as "acute") in RHB hospitals, and these unit costs are applied to acute cases and attendances in Board of Governors hospitals, to give a total for acute hospital services. This leaves a residual expenditure in BG hospitals† (about £90m in 1973/74) which is included in "miscellaneous" hospital expenditure. In addition miscellaneous expenditure includes various other items from the Section 55 and Appropriation Accounts (patients in other hospitals, blood transfusion service, mass radiography, RHB and family practitioner administration, income and various accounting adjustments). Hospital capital expenditure is split on the basis of the special returns for geriatric, mental handicap and mental illness schemes.

6. When expenditure has been allocated to different activities or services in this way for each year, trends in current expenditure are calculated; the results for 1970/71 to 1973/74 are set out in Tables 1 and 2. In addition, an analysis is made wherever possible of how far these trends are due to changes in the level of activity (numbers of cases, places etc.) and how far to changes in unit cost. The analysis suggests that in all hospital services and in local authority residential and day care unit costs have been rising substantially, and account for a significant proportion of the increase in expenditure. This may be due to new, more expensive methods of treatment, the higher proportion of elderly in-patients who need more nursing care, higher standards including higher staffing levels, possibly some wage drift (eg changes in seniority, grade structure

---

* Summaries of the hospital costing returns are published annually by HMSO, but they will not be published for 1974/75.
† Some allowance is made for the different case mix in BG hospitals by costing different groups of acute specialties through a regression analysis.

and overtime which are not allowed for in the wage and salary indices) and some fall in the real level of charges for local authority services.

7. The latest available accounting information is for 1973/74, and, since the HPSS are moving from a period of substantial growth into one of lower growth, it is essential to make an estimate of the position likely to be reached in 1975/76. For family practitioner and centrally financed services, Departmental estimates are available. For current expenditure on hospitals and community health services, trends in 1972/73 to 1973/74 (these are broadly similar to trends over a longer period) are extrapolated for a further two years, but with an adjustment so that the total matches the public expenditure total. For capital expenditure estimates are again based on the public expenditure survey total, and use the latest returns of geriatric, psychiatric and health centre expenditure. For personal social services, the projections start from an estimate of the position likely to be reached in 1976/77, based on the Rate Support Grant negotiations.

8. From the 1975/76 or 1976/77 base, an estimate is then made of the cost of policies for the development of each group of services. In the case of the family practitioner services and welfare food, this is a forecast based on expected demand. For other services, estimates are based on a whole range of considerations, eg specific policies on provision for the mentally ill and handicapped and children in care, the impact of demography, the effects of recent legislation, and general priorities, eg for community care. The costs are then brought together and compared with the overall constraint on public expenditure on health and personal social services as set out in the Public Expenditure White Paper. Priorities are then considered and estimates revised to a level of development compatible with this total. Among the important issues raised in considering priorities is the minimum rate of development at which a policy remains viable, and the point at which a complete change of strategy may become necessary.

9. Working sheets summarising the analysis up to 1975/76 and projections up to 1979/80 at a level of expenditure compatible with the Public Expenditure White Paper, are attached at Tables 1 and 2. In Table 2, the proposed expenditure of £27m by NHS authorities on local authority services under joint financing arrangements is shown under local authority services. Expenditure totals are shown to the nearest £1m because further rounding significantly distorts relative growth rates, but *it cannot be stressed too strongly that the figures are not accurate to this extent. The projections are presented as a quantitative illustration of the priorities put forward* in this document; they are not a detailed plan. The priorities are themselves still subject to consultation, but even if they are not if would be quite impossible to plan to this degree of accuracy this far ahead at a national aggregate level.

10. In addition to this general warning, the following specific points should be borne in mind in interpreting the figures. In relation to past expenditure, one important assumption is that geriatric, psychiatric and maternity patients in acute hospitals cost the same as in special hospitals—in particular only a third of maternity cases are in Type 11 hospitals. However, the estimates for future years are not very sensitive in aggregate to errors in allocation of costs in the base year. The important point is that all expenditure is counted once in the

80

base year, and if some is allocated to the wrong "box", the only effect in aggregate is that a different growth rate is applied to this misallocated sum. In a period of rapid inflation, estimates of past expenditure at constant prices are highly sensitive to errors in the estimates of wage and price changes. In making estimates of future expenditure, two sensitive assumptions are that there will be no further wage drift and that current unit costs for local authority residential and day care can in future be held constant; this implies that standards will not be improved and that charges will rise as fast as costs. There is also considerable uncertainty about some capital unit costs, especially for hospital provision. Nevertheless, it is felt that the figures are sufficiently accurate for a broad exploration of priorities.

11. In addition, the financial projections can be used in considering how resources might be divided between health and personal social services and between capital and current expenditure. Given certain assumptions about relationships between finance and manpower, one can also examine the possible manpower implications of and constraints on proposed expenditure priorities. The relationship of the national aggregate estimates to NHS and local authority planning has still to be explored, but much of the data used is also available at area/county level; the programme budget projections can be translated into average guidelines of provision for a given population by a given date, to assist planners and to provide a basis for comparison between national and local planning. The plans of field authorities will in any case include variations from national averages for many reasons such as varying local needs and priorities and varying capital stock.

SUMMARY TABLE BY PROGRAMME (£m NOVEMBER 1974 PRICES)

	Average current growth pa 1970/71-1973/74 per cent	1973/74 Outturn Capital £m	1973/74 Outturn Current £m	1975/76 Provisional Estimate Capital £m	1975/76 Provisional Estimate Current £m	1979/80 Illustrative Projection Capital £m	1979/80 Illustrative Projection Current £m	Illustrative average current growth pa 1975/76-1979/80 per cent
GRAND TOTAL	4·3	528	3,630	424	3,992	304	4,332	2·1
PRIMARY CARE Sub-total	1·7	23	648	24	718	18	833	3·8
General Medical Services	1·9		209		223		249	2·8
General Dental Services	−1·9		120		129		139	1·9
General Ophthalmic Services	−8·5		19		24		27	3
Pharmaceutical Services	3·3		276		312		382	5·2
Health Centres(1)	25·2	23	2	24	3	18	5	11
Prevention	5·5		15		15		17	3
Family Planning	66·6		7		12		14	4
GENERAL AND ACUTE HOSPITAL AND MATERNITY SERVICES Sub-total	3·7	300	1,572	233	1,670	155	1,733	0·9
Acute IP and OP	3·0	} 300	1,161	} 233	1,225	} 155	} 1,574	} 1·2
Ambulances	4·0		75		79			
Miscellaneous Hospital(2)	9·2		174		197			
Obstetric IP and OP	3·9		136		143		133	−1·8
Midwives	−1·1		26		26		26	0
SERVICES MAINLY FOR ELDERLY AND PHYSICALLY HANDICAPPED Sub-total	9·0	96	512	76	593	44	673	3·2
Geriatric IP and OP(3)	5·2	34	195	31	212	28	243	3·5
Non-Psychiatric DP	15·4		6		7		9	5
Home Nursing	5·6		52		59		75	6
Chiropody	9·9		8		9		10	3
Residential Care	9·1	54	117	35	142	15	154	2·0
Home Help	14·8		80		91		98	2
Meals	18·9		8		14		15	2
Day Care	—	8	12	9	17	1	20	4
Aids, Adaptations, Phones, etc.	—		9		12		17	9
Services for the Disabled	8·9		25	1	30		32	1·5
SERVICES FOR THE MENTALLY HANDICAPPED Sub-total	8·0	32	167	29	189	25	211	2·8
Mental Handicap IP and OP	6·6	14	136	12	146	9	156	1·6
Residential Care	17·0	9	10	9	15	10	20	7
Day Care	—	9	21	8	28	6	36	6·5
SERVICES FOR THE MENTALLY ILL Sub-total	3·6	28	303	23	320	36	344	1·8
Mental Illness IP and OP	3·0	23	280	17	291	25	306	1·3
Psychiatric DP	14·5		10		13		16	5
Residential Care	12·6	2	3	2	4	3	5	7
Day Care	—	1	3	2	4	4	7	15
Special Hospitals	5·6	2	7	2	8	4	10	6
SERVICES MAINLY FOR CHILDREN Sub-total	0·5	16	232	22	266	13	290	2·2
Clinics	2·9		25		26		26	0
Health Visiting	2·5		33		34		43	6
School Health	7·3		48		51		51	0
Welfare Food	−44·6		8		8		8	0
Residential Care	16·7	12	84	18	110	10	121	2·5
Boarding Out	8·4		12		14		15	2
Day Nurseries	7·2	3	17	3	20	1	22	2·5
Central Grants and YTCs	−18·2	1	5	1	3	1	4	6
OTHER SERVICES Sub-total	11·0	33	196	17	236	13	248	1·2
Social Work	11·0		88		105		114	2
Additional Social Services Training	—		—		—		6	—
Other LA Services(4)	—	24	18	14	23	9	23	0
Miscellaneous Centrally Financed Services(5)	17·3	9	90	3	108	4	105	− 0·8

Rounding: Illustrative growth rates 1975/76 to 1979/80 are generally rounded to the nearest 1 per cent pa, except where expenditure exceeds £100m. *All figures are approximate.* Discrepancies due to rounding.

Abbreviations: IP, OP, DP, YTCs—in-patients, out-patients, day patients, youth treatment centres.

(1) Capital figures include expenditure on clinics and other community health.

(2) Includes extra costs of teaching hospitals, RHB and FP administration (pre-reorganisation), mass radiography, blood transfusion services, income and accounting adjustments.

(3) Includes units for the younger disabled.

(4) Includes capital expenditure on land, vehicles, etc.

(5) Includes other health expenditure, Departmental administration and research.

SUMMARY TABLE BY SECTOR (£m NOVEMBER 1974 PRICES)

	Average current growth pa 1970/71-1973/74 per cent	1973/74 Outturn Capital £m	Current £m	1975/76 Provisional Estimate Capital £m	Current £m	1979/80 Illustrative Projection Capital £m	Current £m	Illustrative average current growth pa 1975/76-1979/80 per cent
GRAND TOTAL	4·3	528	3,630	424	3,992	304	4,332	2·1
HOSPITAL AND COMMUNITY HEALTH Sub-total	4·2	394	2,389	317	2,548	235	2,703	1·5
Acute IP and OP	3·0	} 300	1,161	} 233	1,225	} 155	} 1,574	} 1·2
Ambulances	4·0		75		79			
Miscellaneous Hospital(1)	9·2		174		197			
Obstetric IP and OP	3·9		136		143		133	— 1·8
Geriatric IP and OP(2)	5·2	34	195	31	212	28	243	3·5
Non-Psychiatric DP	15·4		6		7		9	5
Mental Handicap IP and OP	6·6	14	136	12	146	9	156	1·6
Mental Illness IP and OP	3·0	23	280	17	291	25	306	1·3
Psychiatric DP	14·5		10		13		16	5
Health Centres(3)	25·2	23	2	24	3	18	5	11
Clinics	2·9		25		26		26	0
Health Visiting	2·5		33		34		43	6
Home Nursing	5·6		52		59		75	6
Midwives	— 1·1		26		26		26	0
Prevention	5·5		15		15		17	3
Chiropody	9·9		8		9		10	3
Family Planning	66·6		7		12		14	4
School Health	7·3		48		51		51	0
FAMILY PRACTITIONER SERVICES Sub-total	1·3		624		688		797	3·7
General Medical Services	1·9		209		223		249	2·8
General Dental Services	— 1·9		120		129		139	1·9
General Ophthalmic Services	— 8·5		19		24		27	3
Pharmaceutical Services	3·3		276		312		382	5·2
LA PERSONAL SOCIAL SERVICES(4) Sub-total	12·2	122	482	100	599	59	673	2·9
Residential: Elderly and Disabled	9·1	54	117	35	142	15	154	2
Mental Handicap	17·0	9	10	9	15	10	20	7
Mental Illness	12·6	2	3	2	4	3	5	7
Children	16·7	12	84	18	110	10	121	2·5
Boarding Out	8·4		12		14		15	2
Home Help	14·8		80		91		98	2
Meals	18·9		8		14		15	2
Day Care: Elderly and Disabled	} 18·5	8	12	9	17	1	20	4
Mental Handicap		9	21	8	28	6	36	6·5
Mental Illness		1	3	2	4	4	7	15
Day Nurseries	7·2	3	17	3	20	1	22	2·5
Aids, Adaptations, Phones, etc.	—		9		12		17	9
Social Work	11·0		88		105		114	2·0
Additional Social Services Training	—		—		—		6	—
Other LA Services(5)	—	24	18	14	23	9	23	0
CENTRALLY FINANCED SERVICES Sub-total	— 1·5	12	135	7	157	10	159	0·3
Welfare Food	— 44·6		8		8		8	0
Services for the Disabled	8·9		25	1	30		32	1·5
Special Hospitals	5·6	2	7	2	8	4	10	6
Central Grants and YTCs	— 18·2	1	5	1	3	1	4	6
Miscellaneous Centrally Financed Services(6)	17·3	9	90	3	108	4	105	— 0·8

Rounding: Illustrative growth rates 1975/76 to 1979/80 are generally rounded to the nearest 1 per cent pa except where expenditure exceeds £100m. *All figures are approximate.* Discrepancies due to rounding.
 Abbreviations: IP, OP, DP, YTCs—in-patients, out-patients, day patients, youth treatment centres.
(1) Includes extra costs of teaching hospitals, RHB and FP administration (pre reorganisation), mass radiography, blood transfusion service, income and accounting adjustments.
(2) Includes units for the younger disabled.
(3) Capital figures include expenditure on clinics and other community health.
(4) Includes development of LA services financed by the NHS under proposed joint financing arrangements.
(5) Includes capital expenditure on land, vehicles, etc.
(6) Includes other health expenditure, Departmental administration and research.

Printed in England for Her Majesty's Stationery Office by Galliard (Printers) Ltd, Great Yarmouth
3839 Dd. 290479 K80 6/76 GL.3917